Dilemmas in Modern

GH00733099

Dilemmas in Modern Health Care

edited by John Spiers

The Social Market Foundation
November 1997

First published by The Social Market Foundation, 1997
in association with Profile Books Ltd

The Social Market Foundation
11 Tufton Street
London SW1 3QB

Profile Books Ltd
62 Queen Anne Street
London W1M 9LA

Printed in Great Britain by Watkiss Studios Ltd

A CIP catalogue record for this book is available from the British Library.

Paper No.33

ISBN 1 874097 070

Contents

Contributors

JOHN SPIERS is Health Policy Adviser to the Social Market Foundation. His books include *The Invisible Hospital and the Secret Garden* (1995) and *Who Owns Our Bodies? Making Moral Choices in Health Care* (1996).

IAN WYLIE is Head of Communications at the King's Fund. He is adviser to the Department of International Development and the author of the NHS Confederation *Guide to Good Communications in NHS Trusts* (1997).

ADAM DARKINS is a British trained neurosurgeon, senior manager and researcher, now working in Denver, Colorado. His interests include involving patients in decision-making and how new technologies improve health care delivery.

HOWARD FREEMAN is Vice President of the National Association of Fundholding Practices and a non-executive director of his health authority. His inner London practice is part of a large multi-practice first wave Total Fundholding Pilot.

MARTIN ROBERTS is Chief Executive of Lambeth Southwark and Lewisham Health Authority. His interests include developing primary care services and examining the impact of strategic changes in acute services on the health and social care system.

JOHN RICHARDS is Head of Performance Management and Development at Southampton and South West Hampshire Health Authority. He has written widely on the subject of priority setting.

TONY SHAW is Chief Executive of Southampton and South West Hampshire Health Authority. He is also a member of the National Steering Group on Setting Priorities in Health Care and was awarded an OBE in 1996 for his contributions to the NHS.

SIÂN GRIFFITHS is Director of Public Health and Health Policy for Oxfordshire. She is Treasurer of the Faculty of Public Health Medicine and Co-Chair of the Association of Public Health.

JONATHAN MCWILLIAM is a consultant in Public Health Medicine in Oxfordshire Health Authority. His interests include developing health policy at the interface of primary and secondary care.

Foreword

The National Health Service is one of Britain's most cherished and important institutions. However it is also first and foremost an organisation charged with delivering better quality care to more people under continuing financial restraint. This has created an ongoing pressure for the NHS service to adapt to the changing world around it and has raised some intriguing dilemmas which we will all have to grapple with as patients, clinicians, managers or business people. Representatives from all these groups contributed chapters here which outline these dilemmas and discuss openly how they might be resolved or at least mediated.

This has been a collaborative exercise. Historically, the relationship between the British pharmaceutical industry and its main customer, the NHS, has been one of mutual dependence tempered by a degree of scepticism. To a certain extent that description could apply to relations between all the authors but *Dilemmas in Modern Health Care* reflects the spirit of co-operation and a willingness to think beyond the normal bounds which will be essential if the NHS is to face the future with confidence.

What emerges is a body of work which we hope will promote a wider understanding of the factors which lie behind the different challenges the NHS faces: one which will accord with the everyday experiences of health professionals;

address itself to their concerns; and also inform a wider public about what is at stake when we talk about the future of the NHS. Above all we hope that *Dilemmas in Modern Health Care* will challenge some conventional thinking and provoke further discussion on what is one of the most important issues of our time.

Ken Moran
Chairman and Managing Director
Pfizer Limited
November 1997

Introduction

John Spiers

It was once said of Prince de Talleyrand – perhaps the subtlest of all policy thinkers – that 'there was this advantage with him, that no question surprised him, and that the most unexpected ones pleased him the best'.[1] It is in this spirit that the Social Market Foundation and Pfizer Limited recently held a series of seminars on modern health care dilemmas to identify the key fault lines in health policy and the options for change. We invited speakers to identify the main challenges confronting us, to suggest possible alternative solutions and to outline the incentives required to bring these solutions about. That task has become all the more intriguing since the new Labour government declared itself open to a complete review of 'hard choices'.

What emerges throughout this paper is that the chief dilemma is political: how to reconcile the underlying principle of the NHS – assuring equal access to health care for all – with a more open approach to competition, which will empower the consumer. This will require a new approach, one which links compassion with markets. It will need a strong economy which can carry health costs without being undermined by them. And it will demand a system capable of providing opportunities, while at the same time protecting those ill equipped to take them. A greater use of markets may not be the whole answer, but neither is abandoning them altogether. We need to retain what is best about the NHS, the public commitment to its epic and intimate qualities, while addressing its shortcomings in terms of quality of care and choice. This means supporting competition between hospitals and practitioners while retaining the support of the public.[2]

It also means mapping out a reform strategy which unites the founding values of the NHS with the potential for individual responsibility; a way of channelling information to, and from, patients and translating this into knowledge which enables people to act through the financial leverage provided by choice. The alternative is what we have today – a system which encourages people to be ignorant and one where the struggle to function within budgets and to emphasise the values of the 1940s has become self-defeating. Robbed of alternative methods of finance and of other sources of expertise, the NHS is now failing to fulfil the most important of these values: equity has been undermined.[3]

The authors of the six following chapters are insiders, encouraged to consider policy in light of a society which has changed drastically since the launch of the NHS fifty years ago. In all of the chapters, rationing is highlighted as a common cause of the problems which face the NHS today.

The rationing debate

Rationing is now widely admitted to be a fact of life in the NHS, but the unpriced system for allocating resources, inherited from the 1940s, hides the relative cost of alternative services and suppliers. It prevents individuals expressing preferences based on individual wishes on the resources available, timing, location, choice of surgeon, treatment, facilities, preferred outcome, care-plan and any additional benefits people seek and would pay for.

Rationing is inextricably linked to outcomes. The analysis of outcomes seeks to isolate the effects of a particular intervention on the health status of either an individual or a whole population. Freeman and Roberts in Chapter 3 examine the complexities of health outcomes and the rationing problems of public health policy. They do so at a time when the gap between demands on the NHS and the resources available is widening, and when the ability to bridge that gap through efficiency gains is decreasing. One consequence of this is the denial of effective care to some patients, notably some of those in terminal decline. Freeman and Roberts probe the apparent conflict between the government's public commitment to a universal NHS and its financial objectives and suggest possible ways out.

It is a theme which Wylie focuses on in Chapter 1. The NHS faces constant pressure to constrain costs in the midst of a culture of medical and scientific innovation which creates new and seemingly limitless demand. Traditionally, health authorities have performed a utilitarian role: providing the greatest amount of 'care' to assure the greatest 'benefit' to the most people. As Wylie shows, that role will be challenged if public policy moves towards more patient choice and with it the likelihood of higher spending. Existing funding structures will inevitably have to change. To say that the health service needs more money is to state the problem but not the solution.[4] Yet, as Wylie says, health budgets may need to grow by 3 per cent each year for the NHS to sustain even present levels of care.

How, then, can more funding be generated, and who is best placed to identify preferences and priorities? The only solution may be for individuals to ration themselves. Wylie hints at this:

Giving patients the facts allows them to decide for themselves the trade-off [in rationing decisions] that only they can make. It puts the clinicians where they should be as advisers and servants of patients, and allows an equity of relationship which is essential to health care: the clinician with specialist knowledge of one sort, the patient with specialist knowledge of another'. (p. 30)

He lays bare the roots of inevitable rationing in health care, considering (but dismissing) the argument that explicit rationing can be avoided by modest increases in expenditure and more efficiency. He is surely equally realistic in saying that no society on a collectivist basis will ever be able to offer every citizen access to every effective treatment whenever it is needed. Thus, anything less is inevitably a trade-off. But who is to make the trade-offs? Wylie's preferred solution is to inform people fully about options, costs, resources, benefits and outcome measures, but not to give them money. There is some evidence that shows informed individuals making different, and cheaper, trade-offs than clinicians. But they do so without a cost-conscious personal budget, they may insist on services irrespective of the financial limitations imposed by government. What happens then?

Mental health

A considerable (and morally difficult) dilemma arises when the criteria for discharging patients from care and treatment are considered. As Freeman and Roberts point out in Chapter 3, there is no contract between the NHS patient and the clinical professional, save for the service-user in mental health care. Individuals only discover service limitations when they seek to enter, or remain within, the system. They ask why a contract should be acceptable in the treatment of mental health, but not in other areas? If the patient is to comply then why not the professional? We come back again to asking what would the necessary incentives be. The exclusion of some patients from treatments is increasingly based on professional judgements of clinical effectiveness. But this, as they argue, posits those dilemmas about the nature and quality of the evidence, which Darkins considers in Chapter 2.

In Chapter 5, Turner analyses mental health care in community settings. This opens up many issues that have been largely hidden from the general public and underestimated by professionals. In urban settings, the problems of failure are increasingly visible and stressful. He looks at the effect this has had on community, responsibility, outcomes, the revision of professional boundaries and the use of financial incentives to achieve sensitised objectives. He shows that while most mental health patients lead 'quietly uninteresting lives' (even if the media often dramatise unrepresentative cases) and that most tasks are mundane in terms of continuing care, the issues themselves are dramatic.

Turner addresses the disparate, complex, politically charged nature of mental health care in community settings. It is in seeking to provide care in the community that some of the most worrying deficits of the existing system are most clearly seen. And, as he shows, there are significant barriers that prevent specific benefit for patients – including nimbyism, discrimination, financial shortages, homelessness and transience, stress on carers and deficits in respite care and after-care.

In mental health care the patient is more than usually isolated. In Turner's view, personal freedom in one's style of living is the essence of community care and positive incentives must be provided to realise this. If real change and significant benefit to patients is to be achieved, resources sufficient for the complex and challenging tasks must be linked to incentives. Again, creative innovation in funding is wanted; for example, local tax-credits for communities accepting hostels for mentally disordered offenders and those involved in voluntary work.

A critical dilemma is how to co-ordinate social and health services. The main barriers here are professional, managerial and political. Yet the idea of community care for the mentally ill necessitates that health and social care are one and indivisible. This is the framework within which the problems of rising expectations and community stigmatism can be tackled. In Turner's analysis, voluntary care and a genuine sense of community have essential roles to play in any solution offered.

Power relationships

In Chapters 4 and 6, Richards and Shaw, Griffiths and McWilliam see rationing as a professional responsibility at the local level, especially at the interface between primary and secondary care. They believe health care will be improved by professionals and managers. They see the greatest gains from the 'empowerment and mobilisation of primary care' by Locality Commissioning, which will enable rationing to be conducted more effectively by the GP — whose offices, note, retain the culturally odd but metaphorically powerful title of 'surgeries'. There are, of course, very significant difficulties about primary care. We know too little about what goes on there. Within this structure, incentives are necessary for the GP to become a networker of networks and assist patients in making their own choices.

One response to the vision of health authority development might be to say that GPs, as purchasers of services, ought to understand the benefit of patients having the financial clout and information which health authorities have recently enjoyed. They, who have experienced the benefits of having the power to make some real changes themselves, should understand why individual patients, and user-groups, might now want the same. Otherwise, there remains an anxiety about the belief in planning as the resolution of health care dilemmas, and a concern about over-reliance on professional judgement. Doctors and patients need to negotiate with each other, considering together any uncertainties or course of action the patient prefers.

The most radical change would be if individuals could choose between providers, who would sustain themselves by excelling competitors in terms of their quality, customer care, environment, prompt access and continuing care. This idea, as Richards and Shaw acknowledge, calls into question whether the NHS should hold 'ownership' of the provision of health care. This is surely not inevitable. Provision could be offered by any organisation that meets government standards and can sustain itself within the market. The question then is: do we want an improved version of the NHS or a different model entirely?

Evidence and choice

'Outcomes' and 'evidence-based medicine' have become buzz-words of today. In Chapter 2 Darkins examines evidence-based medicine (EBM), which exposes the quality of current practice and professional relationships to outside scrutiny. This is starkly illustrated by the fact that only around 20 per cent of interventions are of proven effectiveness. And, like Wylie, Darkins looks at the general dilemmas regarding the ownership of decision-making in health care.

Darkins probes within, questioning 'expertise' and clarifying quandaries about empowerment and quality. He asks whose evidence and preferences should form the basis of decisions about individual lives. In posing these questions, he suggests that the task is to change what counts as evidence, especially in the face of significant evidential uncertainty and the social bias of much public health. In his answers, he shows that there is no clear and recognised process to ensure that the wants of patients are at least included (if no more than that) in clinical decision-making. Darkins, trained as a brain surgeon, offers a different perspective from the health service manager. He is accustomed to addressing the problems of the specific patient in front of him, rather than the 'needs' of a theoretical putative 'population'. Having looked at what happens to specific patients, he is concerned with the whole culture of health care professionals and examines its impact on patient benefit and patient-defined outcomes.

His is a report from 'inside the citadel', offering an unusual trinity: the focus on patient benefit; sensitivity to professional concerns and an awareness of the political dimensions. He rigorously emphasises, again, the problem of incentives. In the NHS, there are no clear incentives to control costs, define and monitor quality, ensure that services are maintained, measure effectiveness, relate the professional activity to the patient, or to assess the patient outcomes from the process. Usually, too, institutional solutions are offered for structures which themselves institutionalise unattractive practice.

Darkins targets the dilemmas of EBM, revealing the unreliability of standards and the intellectual and cultural basis of surprising variations in clinical practice. He tells us that the larger part of health care is not based on rigour and rationality, which calls into question many assumptions as to what the NHS has achieved in routine treatments over the past fifty years. Is it the best in the world? How do we judge and how do we know how we measure up? The ambiguities were barely noticed for a long time in the busy round of daily practice. Thus, many years elapse between a demonstrably harmful treatment and its abandonment by all practitioners. Yet by 1997, evidence-based medicine has become a significant response by clinicians and managers to health service renovation. It may not be the salvation commonly supposed, unless it is itself co-opted by arguments about the values of the individual and the challenges of empowerment which will privilege patient autonomy.

Most critically, Darkins is concerned with the redefinition of EBM and its value from multiple perspectives. This includes the ethical and procedural basis of clinical trials from which practice guidelines derive. He places these issues in a wider context than the everyday assumptions of hospital-based practitioners, and the notion that EBM alone is a buttress to purchasing and practice. He insists that the patient is the fulcrum of care, preferring the phrase 'evidence-based choice' to 'evidence-based practice'. Moreover, he commends evidence-based choice in all clinical practice, not just 'medical' practice.

The challenge of old age

Some of our greatest social dilemmas concerns old age. In Chapter 6, Griffiths and McWilliam tackle the mass of difficulties and dilemmas, trade-offs and compromises, concerning the elderly and social care. This is a heterogeneous and changing group. The authors look at the demographic and epidemiological factors which place the issue of elderly care – and the care of the elderly carers themselves – in the foreground. These include the controversial issues of moral choice at the end of an individual's life, also identified by Wylie, Freeman and Roberts as unsatisfactory areas of present public policy.

Improvements in acute care enable more people to survive into older age, which is characterised by chronic and disabling conditions. Chronic diseases are isolating. They set the patient apart and are a major strain on the suffering individual, their families and resources. By their nature, they are long-term and uncertain in prognosis. They often raise multiple problems which call for a range of services, including home care. This imposes enormous demand on carers and budgets, as shown by the increasing claims for GP services to operate on a 24-hour basis as well as for institutional care. The challenge is significant for the individual, the carer and the state.

In the NHS, constraints on resources require rationing based on what Griffiths and McWilliam call 'objective clinical criteria'. These choices become more harrowing as costly new treatments offer new therapies for previously untreatable conditions. Once again, the issue is 'who decides who decides?' Who pays for treatments and choices, and how? How are objective criteria to be legitimised and subjective criteria to be empowered? How is social sanction to be secured for health authority plans, for example, for denying renal services by age and post-code? As the NHS becomes more explicitly a safety net service, especially for the young and the elderly, in which areas of health care is the state prepared to turn people away?

The patient always pays

Ultimately, it is always the patient who takes the risks, in all health care interventions. This underlies all health care dilemmas. It shows that patient benefit should be the object of all exercises. Ultimately, we are all responsible for ourselves and for our own individual lives and bodies. The fact that the patient takes the risks intrudes uniquely upon every relationship, especially in the decision-making process between doctor and patient. Financial structures should enable the successful delivery of individual, separable patient benefit. This should focus all health care providers on the one sustainable advantage: organisational consciousness and learning for patient benefit. The objective is to achieve proven quality outputs which individuals want as they actively cope in their own terms with their own challenges.

It is often necessary to reconcile paradoxical agendas. This requires both the professional and the patient to be effectively engaged so that we can discover what really goes on in relationships and transactions in health care, how to openly listen and how to act for change. Voting does not secure this: economics may. Health care purchasing – with existing NHS providers perhaps established as local charities – must be closely orientated around individual patients. Patients are the source of special and unique knowledge in a democracy, rather than the recipients of the special role that 'expert' knowledge ought to play. This calls for the political finesse of high-grade change management to realise the power of the patient's preference and experience. This is, indeed, the essential link and context for different kinds of expertise, and the necessary protection for deep cultural diversity.

Thus, as these dilemmas become more explicit, a cultural policy will be required to discipline the aims of public policy. Meanwhile, the problems of financing, rationing, defining quality and the management of professionals remain.

These policy debates are not, however, only about the NHS. When we speak of the dilemmas of health care we do not refer of the NHS alone, despite the principle of legitimacy to which a near-monopoly NHS appeals in the British psyche. There is a successful and growing private sector (and many public or private partnerships) in Britain. For example, the private sector now provides the majority of elderly care beds. Total independent health care expenditure in 1995 was at least £15 billion on health and social care services. It accounted for three-quarters of the numbers of bed-nights of long-term care (148 million out of 196 million), and its volume of surgical procedures grew from just under 300,000 in 1981 to nearly 750,000 in 1995. Private sector capital investment is also large; for example, some £11,144 million is invested in long-term care.⁵

The health care and cultural dilemmas that this book addresses are inevitably a problem for politics. Here, Talleyrand has the last word. He said that politicians cannot successfully refuse for too long what the age proclaims to be necessary. They must listen to the people:

> There is someone who is cleverer than Voltaire, cleverer than Bonaparte, cleverer than any of the Directors, than any Minister in the past or in the future; and that person is everybody [*tout le monde*]. To engage, or at least to persist, in a struggle in which you may find everybody interested on the other side is a mistake, and nowadays all political mistakes are dangerous.⁶

1. The Cost of Caring: A Tale of Innocence and Experience

Ian Wylie

What is the price of experience? Do men buy it for a song,
Or wisdom for a dance in the street?
William Blake

In July 1997 the argument about euthanasia, which had been a rumbling background noise in Britain for a couple of years, dramatically intensified and became front page news in all the newspapers. The British Medical Association (BMA), at its annual conference in July, had voted decisively against a motion calling for the legalisation of voluntary euthanasia for certain terminal conditions. The decision infuriated two doctors who each publicly admitted that on many occasions they had, with the consent of the patients and close relatives, terminated the lives of people in their care. In each case, they explained, the patient was terminally ill, incapacitated, in pain and living had become unbearable for them. The row escalated. The BMA accused the doctors of playing God, and called for them to be investigated by the police and, if necessary, charged. The doctors retaliated by saying that on occasions the nature of their work required them to act as God, and accused the BMA of rank hypocrisy.[7] Notable in its absence in this argument was the voice of the patient, the so-called informed decision-maker, on whose behalf both sides claim to be acting, and whose interests both claim to defend.

One of the arguments against voluntary euthanasia is the spectacle it conjures of the dying process. Opponents believe that legalising such measures would open up the possibility of terrible abuse; some future government could require the incapacitated, the terminally ill or the very old, to be denied health care and gently dispatched once they had become an intolerable burden on the state. In this scenario, euthanasia becomes a method of controlling the costs of health care by limiting expenditure on those groups – the elderly or terminally ill – which place the greatest burden on the health budget. They cite an article by a senior health economist in the *British Medical Journal* which argues for the concept of a 'fair innings' for older people – suggesting they be denied care when health resources are scarce – and claim it is evidence that their fears are legitimate.[8]

In 1998 the National Health Service will be in its fiftieth year. Almost without exception, the amount that Britain has spent on the NHS has increased in real terms every year since 1948. Conventional economic wisdom suggests that the health budget should grow by 3 per cent each year for the NHS to remain capable of delivering care. Each year expensive new therapies become available to the health service, and as the health of the population improves, people live longer, consume more health resources and expect more from the health service. On its fiftieth anniversary, the health service is facing a period of unparalleled restrictions to its budget while the cost of caring continues to rise.

The legacy of the past fifty years – costs and spending rising inexorably, pressure for even more health care delivery, periodic crises in the health service leading to hospital closures, strikes and severe limits on care – is very different from the future envisaged by the founders of the NHS in 1948. Its architects anticipated a rush of demand in the early years of the NHS as universal provision brought with it a flood of people with health care needs that the pre-1948 system had failed. However, they also believed that after this initial period, and as increased affluence improved the health of the nation, spending on health would gradually decrease.[9] In its fiftieth year there is a very real chance that the costs of caring will outstrip available resources and a danger that the NHS will no longer be able to uphold its claim to provide universal health care, free at the point of delivery, based on need alone.

The row over euthanasia illustrates how fears are growing that health care may be withdrawn from one or more groups of the population, with the consequent loss of provision for all. Advocacy groups for older people argue that this is already happening. Most people will also recognise that access to care which is free at the point of delivery was abandoned long ago in dentistry, drugs and eye care. Although medical care remains free at delivery, the present government has refused to rule out the notion of charges for some services in the future. Most people, however, retain the belief that, most of the time, health care providers in the NHS give individuals the best treatment possible, based solely on the health care needs of individuals.

The idea that health care is rationed and that further rationing is inevitable, is fiercely opposed by some in the medical profession.[10] Yet in a system of limited health care provision and unrestrained demand, it would be strange if there were not some means of limiting the distribution of benefit. In fact, rationing occurs throughout the NHS on the basis of a system of collective and individual decisions about the size and distribution of health care resources. It begins with the government deciding the level of spending from taxation income, and the distribution of NHS resources throughout the country; it extends into the distribution of resources to the several kinds of health care providers, which is guided by decisions on investment in different treatments made by managers and clinical budget holders; and it ends with the individual clinician's judgment on which of the limited treatment options available to use.[11] These constraints on caring are usually tacit and unchallenged. Although they are rarely immoral, they tend not to be based on principle. Indeed, the idea of rationing undermines the NHS's third founding principle, that care is provided solely on the basis of need.

In 1937 Douglas Jay, who was later to become a senior minister in Harold Wilson's government, asserted that 'in the case of nutrition and health, just as in the case of education, the gentlemen in Whitehall really do know better what is good for the people than the people know themselves'.[12] As Lord Jay, he lived long enough both to hear the howl of complaint when 'democracy was removed from the NHS' and local government lost the right to appoint councillors to NHS boards, and also to witness the rise of consumer power in public services with local and national service charters.

As expectations have increased, so the rhetoric has changed. When the NHS began to involve the public in decisions about services, both collectively and individually, 'customer service' was replaced by 'patient empowerment' and, more recently, by 'patient partnership'. New ways of consulting the public on service planning have been piloted with Citizens' Juries, where a panel of community representatives takes evidence from expert witnesses before making their recommendations for investment and disinvestment.[13] In planning and providing individual services, health authorities and NHS Trusts regularly consult a wide variety of specialist interest groups, voluntary experts, users' panels, market research companies and individual patients and carers. At the level of individual care, offering an informed choice between several treatment options has become the gold standard, with the patient fully involved in decisions with the clinician.[14]

So what is the problem? Let us begin with the idea of informed decision-making. As John Spiers has persuasively shown,[15] it will soon be quite common for patients to come to a consultation, even with a consultant specialist, knowing more about the latest research findings on treatment for their condition from an Internet web site than the specialist. What these patients will certainly not know are the budgetary constraints under which their specialist is operating, such as spending targets for drug or technical therapies; the clinical priorities which have placed that specialty in a relative scale of importance; the needs assessment profile of the resident population to establish the resource allocation and health priorities for the year; or even the research funded by drug companies on which the specialist relies to fund the department. All these will be deciding factors in the treatment options available to the patient. If the specialist agrees to a patient's request to be treated with the latest expensive therapy, will the next patient be told this? Is it relevant? We cling naïvely to the view that it is not, and that each patient is treated solely on the evidence presented. But if the budget will allow only five patients to receive a particular therapy, what will happen to the sixth? Patient partnership is not an equal partnership but rather the relationship of a senior to a junior partner. Would the outcomes be improved if the clinician were to admit that the choices available to the patient were limited from the start by cost, previous choices and the clinician's own experience?

There is a further limitation to the patient's freedom of choice. How does the patient know whether the clinician is actually any good? There is virtually no available information for patients on the quality of health care provided by either individual professionals or institutions. No data is published on clinical performance although a large amount is collected. Performance league tables by hospital are published, yet there are no figures on the performances that really matter: how well the hospital cares for its patients. Patients can find out more about the quality of the plumber called in to mend a tap, than the quality of the health provider responsible for their lives. In a system which still does not distinguish between patients who leave hospital alive or dead, we should not be surprised that there are no figures to distinguish a centre of excellence from one of mediocrity.

Perhaps it is as well that we do not. Centres of excellence are expensive to run. Once such centres were widely known, surely everyone would choose to use them? This would mean costs would rise, transport needs would increase and 'sink' centres, deprived of income, would become redundant. These catastrophic consequences on the cost of caring would be the result of rational, informed choices by individual patients, acting within the bounds of the individual's right to choose a particular institution and individual to provide their care.

It was one of the freedom cries of the 1991 changes to the NHS that money should be allowed to follow the patient. This was one of the founding principles on which the division between the purchasing or commissioning of health care and the provision of health care was built. Health authorities were to keep their budgets flexible to allow choice. This has not happened. Indeed, the experience of health authorities is that patient choice, expressed as extra-contractual referrals, is an expensive business, involving special payments to the individually chosen provider as well as the existing block payment to the health authority's preferred provider. So health authorities, which have the utilitarian job of achieving the greatest amount of health care to provide the greatest benefit to the most people, may always be at odds with the notion of individual patient choice.

The utilitarian dilemma was most clearly illustrated in the infamous case of Jaymee Bowen, Child B, a young girl with acute myeloid leukemia.[16] When Cambridge and Huntingdon health authority refused to pay for an experimental treatment, based on the low chances of success, her father went to the High Court to challenge the decision. The tabloid press responded by arguing that while there is life there is hope: any treatment, however small the chance of success, is worthwhile to save a child's life.

Here the contradictions between individualist and collectivist solutions were most graphically, emotively and tragically illustrated. The premature death of any child in the end is a tragedy, both personal and to society. But would that child's death be any more or less tragic if it occurred after several hundred thousand pounds of public resources had been spent, money which would then not be available for effective patient care? Would it be more or less tragic if it occurred after the patient's and father's informed choice to go ahead with treatment carried out by the NHS?

In its fiftieth year, the NHS is impaled on the horns of a dilemma. The cry is for patient choice and informed shared decision-making, yet the approach is based on strict utility. Our increasingly limited resources for health care must be carefully distributed, and individual patient choice may inevitably break the carefully brokered settlement. There are three potential ways out of this dilemma: to increase NHS spending and effectiveness sufficiently to satisfy demand without limiting care; to give patients real power to purchase health care directly; and to give patients enough knowledge to make properly informed choices about their care. I shall look at each of these in turn.

Those who oppose the argument for rationing in the NHS, argue that with modest increases in expenditure funded by the Exchequer and the elimination of all ineffective and inefficient treatments, the NHS would be able to provide full care without the need to ration treatments known to be effective. But although the NHS must continue in the quest for efficiency and effectiveness, others argue that it is both counter-intuitive and a denial of the everyday experience of managers and clinicians, to claim that NHS resources could meet all health needs.

The analogy of the road building programme may clarify this. Over the next twenty-five years there will be 8 million more cars on the roads. How many more roads will we need? We could build enough to keep traffic density to the level it is today. This would be possible but expensive, both financially and environmentally. We could build fewer roads and increase density, which would be cheaper but might ruin our transport infrastructure and our economic competitiveness. We could build enough roads to minimise accidents and re-route traffic from all cities, but only by covering the land in concrete and tarmac. In the end, the number of roads we build is dependent on what sort of balance we are prepared to agree as a society.

Similarly we could increase health expenditure so that every citizen could have access to specialist care whenever it was needed, thus requiring round-the-clock availability of specialist teams, and every possible effective treatment available without restriction. We would then have the most effective, comprehensive and accessible health system in the world. Yet the cost to the country would rule out all other public services. Anything less than this is a trade-off, and any trade-off is, by definition, a limiting or rationing of possible benefit, thus disproving the belief that increases in expenditure and efficiency of the NHS would allow full choice.

The argument for giving patients real spending power relies on the idea that markets – real not internal – are the only way of empowering patients, because only through the operation of markets can need be matched to supply at a cost which is affordable. Criticism of the purchaser/provider split in the NHS centres on the idea that the health authority, which is given a budget to buy health care for a defined population, has no obligation to spend this money effectively on behalf of patients, because it has no stake in the outcome. Hence while health authorities may strive to be responsible in their purchasing decisions, there is no mechanism in the system which requires them to be so, and so the market, which could and should regulate the purchaser's behaviour, is not allowed to operate. The solution is to give the purchasing power directly to individuals by giving them an individual budget, weighted to take account of health needs, and allow them to buy health care in the market place.[17] This will ensure the efficiency and effectiveness of competing health care providers, reducing costs and directly empowering the individual. Patients could choose where to go for treatment or decide to invest in other benefits. For example, a terminally ill patient may decide to go on holiday, rather than undergo a course of chemotherapy to prolong life by a few more months.

Proponents of this 'true' empowerment of individuals argue that it combines the best in collectivist and individualist decision-making. It would be for Parliament to decide on the health care settlement (the value of the voucher) but the informed spending power of the individual would ensure both maximum benefit and a cost-price regime which maximised efficiency. Yet, it would also ensure the death of collective responsibility for the health and welfare of individuals. The NHS was founded on the principle of social justice, the equal worth and dignity of every member of society. The idea of individuals negotiating the best deals for themselves from competing providers could not be further from the concept of social justice. The modern welfare state is based on the principle that whatever an individual's ability, circumstances, hopes, fears and character, there are certain basic provisions that society can make collectively and equitably to all. Without these basic values there is no NHS. Thus, the voucher scheme is a solution, but not one which is possible within the constitution of the NHS.

The third way out of the dilemma of utilitarian distribution and individual demand, is to give patients and carers all the information possible about the health care options available, including the cost of treatments, resources, benefits and the performance figures of the health care providers. It is then the decision of the individual alone which option to choose. Patients go into the health service in a state of innocence, knowing next to nothing about the rules – financial, managerial, professional and political – which determine the treatment choices that are made for them. When a clinician says to a patient, 'we have done the best we can', what is meant is 'we have done the best we can do within the limits we are set by the health service'. This is not made explicit. Yet each patient is part of the democratic process that has caused those limits to be set, and only when they know as much as the clinician about the boundaries will they be able to participate fully in their own health care.

This chapter opened by discussing euthanasia and the doctors who are accused of playing God. Yet carrying out the wishes of patients to die in a dignified way at a time and place of their choosing is the role of a servant not a deity. Allowing patients to take an informed decision about their health care is only irreconcilable with the responsibility to achieve maximum health care if patients regularly choose eccentric treatments which do not work but are very costly. Recent research suggests that, in reality, this does not happen. In trials with cancer patients it has been shown that, once presented with the full facts of treatments, outcomes and costs, patients' choices were actually cheaper than those made by the clinicians, because unlike the clinicians, cancer patients were able to trade quality of life for quantity of life and not feel that they had failed.[18] Similarly, for every tragic and newsworthy story of parents' desperate flights across the globe for a life-saving, frontier-breaking treatment for their child, there are countless other parents who face the death of a child by trying to make their last months as happy, rich and pain-free as possible. Giving patients the facts allows them to decide for themselves the trade-off that only they can make. It puts the clinicians where they should be, as advisers and servants of patients, and allows an equality between the two parties which is essential to health care: the clinician with specialist knowledge of one sort, the patient with specialist knowledge of another. This may signal the death of innocence, but care based on experience must be worth the fight.

2. Evidence-based Medicine: A Consensus Dream or a Practical Reality?

Adam Darkins

If, as research indicates, only 20 per cent of current medical practice has evidence of 'effectiveness' to support its use then this is surely scandalous and the situation must change.[19] This seems self-evident. Why, therefore, is there a debate about implementing a programme of evidence-based medicine? The cause, as is so often the case, lies buried in the detail. Although evidence-based medicine is a fine and worthy principal, it is mere 'motherhood and apple pie' unless crucial issues, surrounding both its definition and how it will be implemented, are resolved. This chapter examines these associated problems of definition and implementation, and places evidence-based medicine in a wider perspective: that of the health care system within which it must operate. The answers or solutions offered place the patient at the heart of the health care delivery system, thus focusing not just on evidence-based practice but also on evidence-based choice.

If any sense of rationality underpins our health care systems, there are *de facto* arguments which support basing all clinical practice, not just medical practice, upon evidence of effectiveness. This is because it is crucially the patient, or 'user' of health care services, who ultimately bears the direct risk of undergoing care. Given that any health care intervention has the potential to cause harm, as well as to do good, it follows that they should not be condoned unless they are based on evidence that they 'work'.[20] A necessary caveat to this is when new evidence of efficacy and effectiveness needs to be obtained through scientific trials.

Scientific trials of health care interventions now use guidelines to develop protocols that protect participants from harm. All clinical trials should now have a clearly agreed ethical and scientific framework before they are undertaken. The guidelines from which these frameworks derive are intended to ensure that clinical trials ask valid and reasonable questions that justify the experiment on patients. A necessary part of the ethical and scientific assessment is to clarify in advance the appropriateness of any methodology used, and so ensure that any questions that arise do not infringe the rights of patients. If later, in the course of a trial, the patient is harmed, then mechanisms are included in the trial protocols to ensure the trial is modified, or that it ceases. In all trials patients retain a right of non-participation, which they can exercise without any detriment to their future treatment.

Unfortunately health care systems are not based on rationality. Although clinical trials impose a stringency of behaviour when testing new and unproven treatments, there is no comparable rigorous assessment of the existing treatments used in routine clinical practice. Because health care professionals are accustomed to this ambiguity they can continue to use treatments, or refer patients for treatments that have no evidence of effectiveness.

Worse still, some clinicians continue to use treatments after they are known to be harmful. In the past, for example, radical mastectomy was persistently used to treat breast cancer. It finally ceased to be clinical practice after the pressure initiated by women's groups in America. Women were outraged at this procedure of unnecessary mutilation, as breast cancer surgeons could adopt equally effective, and far less mutilating, treatments for breast cancer. They forced a number of recalcitrant surgeons to reconsider their practice and subsequently abandon this form of treatment. The evidence had been widely known to clinicians since the publication of large-scale clinical studies, yet they still failed to act on the basis of the evidence until public pressure was bought to bear.[21]

The example of breast cancer and radical mastectomy is important because it raises general issues about the ownership of both decision-making and evidence in health care. Western allopathic systems of health care traditionally empower the clinician, usually the doctor, to take a dominant role in the decision-making process, thereby making the clinician the arbiter of what constitutes the evidence. In the current setting it is surely an indictment of our health care systems that although they pride themselves upon the scientific basis of medicine, research shows that only 20 per cent of interventions are of proven effectiveness.[22] Clearly the old conspiracy based on the idea that the 'doctor knows best' remains, and needs to be challenged if evidence-based practice is to develop and become a potent force for organisational change and continued overhaul of our health care systems.

Health care professionals, particularly doctors, traditionally have great latitude and autonomy in their modes of practice, because of the extensive variations in the ways in which care for common conditions is delivered.[23] Until recently standards of clinical decision-making have not been explicitly challenged. Although the needs of patients as individuals change (as do their personal and clinical situations) there is still no clearly recognised process to ensure those needs and circumstances are accounted for in the decision-making of clinicians. Should the principles upon which health care decisions are taken require evidence from patient experience as well as clinical studies? If they do not, evidence-based practice may continue to reflect nuances of professional practice rather than patient outcome.

This is the crux of the dilemma that evidence-based practice poses for health care systems. By its very nature, evidence-based practice explicitly exposes the quality of both current practice and professional relationships to outside scrutiny. In doing so, it promises to change fundamentally relationships in the health care arena and thereby the current status quo, dominated by autonomous health care professionals whose lines of accountability are unclear. In the future, this degree of autonomy will be untenable. A clinician will no longer be shielded from questioning beneath the convenient umbrella of clinical freedom, unless the accountability and line of responsibility on which this clinical freedom is granted are also made explicit. Until this necessary change occurs, health care will continue to be conducted in Britain and America at the discretion of a range of professional groups.

Let us consider the hypothetical consequences if a similar situation existed in manufacturing industry. What if the front-line production workers on the assembly line decide which accessories to place on each car as it arrives? Should it have alloy wheels, a quadraphonic stereo system, a sun-roof and high performance engine specification? All features would be decided by the assembly line worker with no direct recourse to the customer or management, the only limitations imposed on the production worker's activity being the continued supply of basic cars and provision of accessories. How does this analogy correspond to health care? The front-line production workers are predominantly doctors, the cars are patients, and the accessories represent the funding for items of health care service provision. A system such as this is both unmanageable and unsustainable. There are no clear incentives to control costs, monitor quality, ensure that services are maintained, measure effectiveness, relate the professional activity to the patient, or to assess the patient outcomes from the process. Such a system would be in crisis. Is it therefore any wonder that health care systems are now in degrees of crisis?

It was the break up of the Guilds of Craftsmen in Britain during the Middle Ages that gave rise to the manufacturing industries that we know today, including motor manufacture, to develop. We may not wish health care to emulate too closely a manufacturing production process; there are necessarily vital human elements unique to the clinician/patient relationship. However, we expect from the manufacturing process a consistency of procedure and a predictability of outcome that it would be useful to see translated into clinical practice. Many aspects of the restrictive practices and professional demarcation lines that typified and stultified the medieval guilds have their parallels in health care. These are likely to obstruct the adoption of evidence-based practice. Although many may mourn the loss of the craftsman to industry, it is this change that has brought about the wide availability of many goods and services in society today. Would a change in the health care guilds similarly enable wider availability of health care?

In our current health care systems we have delegated the delivery of health care to particular professionals, and yet we have not required them to follow explicit processes. It is not therefore surprising that much of what is provided for us in health care is based upon an act of faith and not on scientific evidence of effectiveness. An inevitable dilemma in the introduction of evidence-based practice is therefore whether the health care professions are capable of regulating themselves, or whether a new societal structure should undertake this role on their behalf in the future.

The advantage of professional self-regulation is that it is likely to be easier and less expensive, avoid major changes to the structural delivery of health care, and should be less upsetting to the general public. It will be easier because professionals can have ownership of the change, and less expensive because it will not require external support systems (see below). It will avoid major structural change because it will merely continue the same system in an adapted form. Because the proponents of this new way of thinking will be professionals already known to the public, people may find it more comfortable to adapt to evidence-based practice. There are, however, also disadvantages. Self-regulation has, for example, clearly failed so far.[24] Similarly, it may be necessary to change the guild system of health care if health care systems based on evidence of effectiveness are to evolve in the future. The health professional structure that we are accustomed to may in itself be a decisive factor in institutionalising practice that is not reliant on evidence.

So, not surprisingly, the role that evidence-based practice will play is inevitably bound up with the future of the health care systems in which it must be incorporated. There is a current movement within health care systems towards considering their services in terms of the impact they make on improving the health of their 'populations'. This same consideration is a likely reason for adopting areas of evidence-based practice in the future. Health care professionals have traditionally focused on the individual patient rather than taking this wider population perspective. Politicians and health care managers may take the wider perspective, but they are also concerned about overall cost and value for money. Patients' views lie somewhere in between these two perspectives. In this situation there is a place for a new societal mechanism to emerge, which monitors and updates the evidence upon which practice is based while working with, without being wholly dependent upon, professional bodies.

A new societal system along these lines may be emerging in the form of the Internet, which has the benefit of open access and enables information to be shared. Much of the information that previously strengthened the power and mystique of clinicians is now becoming available to the lay public on-line. For example, people with HIV/AIDS can now access on-line databases that can at least keep them abreast, if not in advance, of the knowledge base of the clinicians that they encounter for care. Is the pressure for evidence-based practice therefore arising because information that used to be the preserve of professionals is now available to a much wider circle of people? An informed lay public is less likely to accept that the 'doctor knows best', particularly if they have learned from an Internet web site that there is strong evidence to the contrary.

Information is not valuable in and of itself, and may create a dilemma in terms of an information-based anarchy. Could evidence-based practice fall into the turmoil this creates? The main sources of information for patients used to be the health care professional, local informal networks and the media. We are now enmeshed in a global mass of data which raises a number of questions: what is the evidence? whose evidence is right? is there more information out there somewhere, and where should I look? The process of keeping an 'information base' intact and up-to-date so that it is a reliable source for patients and clinicians, is a major unresolved problem in supporting evidence-based practice in the future. Central governments have started to provide 'independent' sources of evidence – through the Patient Outcome Research Teams (PORTS) in America, and the Cochrane Centre and the Effectiveness Bulletins in Britain. But is the role of central government in effectiveness-based practice clear, or is it confused and contradictory?

One attraction to government of evidence-based practice is that, with only 20 per cent of health care interventions proven effective, it may be possible to harness health care expenditure savings by restricting the 80 per cent of unproven interventions. Governments which are wrestling with the task of containing public expenditure, have a mercenary incentive to promote evidence-based practice as a means of rationing care through abolishing what is ineffective. In Britain, the Cochrane Centre in Oxford was part of a government-sponsored initiative to promote evidence-based practice. Once established, it was rapidly accepted that the task was too large, and the penalties of duplicated effort too wasteful, for any one organisation in one country to take on this mammoth task alone. The Cochrane Centre quickly metamorphosed into the Cochrane Collaboration, set up to co-ordinate the many centres in different countries, each funded by their host government.

Clearly there are great advantages, not only for institutions but also for governments, in collaborating on global protocols for the treatment and care of chronic conditions. If this is to be the case, how will developing the evidence be funded, and, more crucially, who will pay? The United Nations is beset with wrangling between countries over its budget payments. Will central governments continue to have a role in evidence-based practice in the future, given that their research funding is already being reduced, or will it be left to the market and to pharmaceutical companies to translate this into disease management? Because we are bound together globally by diseases that have no respect for national boundaries, evidence-based practice will continue to be of international importance. Although many health care systems are grappling with the challenge of introducing evidence-based practice, none has so far achieved a satisfactory model.

It is not clear what system, or mixture of health care systems, will prevail in the future. Paradoxically, given the effort and energy currently being expended on evidence-based practice, there is no strong evidence to support the process of evidence-based practice for a whole health care system. So far, evidence-based practice has taken a disease-based approach. In Britain, Effectiveness Bulletins reviewed the evidence on a range of topics, from grommets in children's ears to the rate of falls among the elderly. Their success in subsequently changing practice in the health care system as a whole is unclear. How does evidence-based practice relate to the process whereby a myriad of decisions are made each day between clinicians and patients within the health care system dynamic? A 'population' approach is valuable to understanding at one level. However, this understanding needs to be tempered by another perspective, that of the processes which govern individual clinical decision-making between clinician and patient.

So, perhaps neither the reasons behind the adoption of an evidence-based practice approach within a health care system, nor even the specific content of the evidence itself, is the key issue. Perhaps the real dilemma in evidence-based practice places the focus back on the individual clinical decision made between clinician and patient. As with so many aspects of contemporary life, it is not the process itself, but how people fit into the process, that is the challenge. Is evidence-based practice intended to be an antidote to the prescriptive approach of a medical model in which patients are told what treatment to have? If so, will it result in a population-based model of evidence-based practice? This may create an equally prescriptive situation, but one which dictates to an entire population instead of just to an individual patient. The net effect on patient/clinician interaction would remain unchanged in the patient's eyes.

What, therefore, is the patient's perspective in relation to evidence-based practice? If a distillation of the vast libraries of accumulated medical research found that only 20 per cent of practice is justified by evidence, then what has this huge literature been concerned with? It does not seem that its predominant concern has been registering patients' views, which have become subordinate to the research needs of clinicians. It may therefore be time to re-evaluate health care provision and to base it upon patients' views of outcomes. Things can look very different from the other side of the examination table.

Let us consider the situation of a forty-eight-year-old man with low back pain, and pain running down the back of his left leg. The pain in his lower back and running down his left leg came on suddenly when he bent and twisted to pick up a golf ball. Despite resting in bed, this pain does not settle. The doctor diagnoses sciatica. This refers to the pain running down the back of the leg in the area supplied by the sciatic nerve. In essence the diagnosis restates the problem but gives it a Latin name. Radiological investigations show a lumber disk that is successfully removed at operation.

All treatment procedures were followed correctly: a patient of the right age, with the right history of symptom development, and the right physical signs on examination, received the right investigations that led to the right operation and removal of the expected pathology. All boxes ticked and a triumph of modern medical care? Unfortunately the man was among the 30 per cent of patients who continue to suffer low back pain and pain running down the leg post-operatively. So, for the patient, the situation is unchanged except he has undergone an operation that did not work.

This example illustrates that there are risks as well as benefits to treatment, and that it is the patient who primarily bears the consequences. No matter how technically good the surgeon, manual dexterity cannot make up for putting the wrong patient on the operating table. Great emphasis is placed in clinical training on establishing a diagnosis and prescribing treatment; less concern is given to weighing the evidence of treatment and matching this to the needs of patients.

Much of the debate over the introduction of evidence-based practice into health care systems is associated with the effect this will potentially have on clinicians. Legitimate concerns are that clinicians will be threatened and that their clinical freedom will be undermined. Although changes to organisations should be sensitively undertaken, there is a question of parity in this situation. If a clinician is practising sub-standard care, then wounded pride is not a justifiable reason to inflict harm on patients. The question of evidence-based practice overlaps with issues such as 'whistle-blowing' and collusion with bad practice. The idea that health care systems adopt set standards of practice links evidence-based practice with the development of systems for clinical audit.

It is not yet clear how evidence-based practice relates to the direct delivery of patient care. Is it a question of the clinician using evidence as a means of reducing health care costs, or is it that the information is used to share decision-making between clinician and patient? In a publicly funded health service it is accepted that health care services are prioritised. Within this framework of prioritisation the clinician can negotiate with the patient in order to decide jointly on the most appropriate treatment. The clinician often has a vast armamentarium at his/her disposal with which to make a decision. Years of training, familiarity with the condition, a personal rapport with other clinicians and a battery of tests to interpret, support the clinician's role in the decision-making. The patient does not have the same level of resources. Is evidence-based practice aimed at empowering the patient as well as the clinician? If it is, how will this process take place in practice?

If evidence about effectiveness is used by the clinician to help the patient to decide on his/her preferred treatment, then this model of providing patient care changes the role of the health care professional. No longer is health care just about the technical clinical role of prescribing a treatment to a patient. The clinician's role extends to decision support and to fitting the treatment to the needs of the patient. Suddenly the concept of evidence-based practice for the clinician becomes one of evidence-based choice for the patient.

The evidence upon which this shared choice is made then needs to be based upon a variety of sources. This must incorporate both clinical evidence about the effectiveness of treatments, and the experiential evidence from patients, from which patient-based outcomes are derived. The prime role of the clinician becomes one of helping the patient to interpret evidence and putting the wide variety of alternative sources of evidence into perspective. The patient can then make an informed decision about the choices available. The ultimate aim is for patients to become discerning consumers, who relate their health to the appropriate use of health care services and to their lifestyle.

In conclusion, there are many dilemmas associated with health care systems adopting evidence-based medicine. These dilemmas relate to the definition of what constitutes evidence-based medicine, and to how this is then implemented. It is important that organisations and health care systems resolve these dilemmas by having a well-defined strategy for adopting evidence-based practice. Defining a strategy requires a clear understanding of what evidence-based health care is intended to achieve. Is it intended to save resources? Is it intended as a quality initiative that fits with clinical audit and standard setting? Is it intended as a means of helping patients make choices about the care they receive? Evidence-based medicine, if adopted, promises to change the culture of health care delivery and become an ongoing commitment.

3: Health Care Funding and Outcomes: Will Your NHS Insurance Cover Meet Your Needs?

Howard Freeman and
Martin Roberts

The NHS Executive defines the aim in health outcomes as 'to secure through the resources available the greatest improvement in the physical and mental health of people in England'.[25] The elegant simplicity of this statement masks its actual complexity. It refers to not just the work of the NHS but also all the partners the NHS works with to influence health. It incorporates all the many single interventions and decisions made by different players as well as the health of individuals and whole populations. It encompasses different perspectives and cultures and the need to collect information from many different systems, some of which currently may not exist. It may be better to think of health outcomes in terms of a definition used by the Central Health Outcomes Unit (CHOU) which was set up as an internal Department of Health Unit in 1993. CHOU defines health outcomes as the 'attributable effect of intervention or its lack on a previous health state'.[26]

The NHS national policy framework seeks to obtain the best possible link between the use of the resources available and improving the health of the population so that evaluating health outcomes becomes a matter of the utilisation of and benefit derived from resources. When evaluating health outcomes, what we are in effect trying to do is to isolate the influence of a particular intervention on the health status of either an individual or a whole population. An aim for the future for the NHS could usefully be that every health care professional within the service understands the effect of each of their interventions on the health outcomes both for that patient and for the broader population.

Since 1993, Population Health Outcome Indicators have been available. They are published annually and reflect population health endpoints (morbidity, mortality, interventions as proxies) for conditions where the NHS has an implicit contributory role. Changes in the public health common data are set to include environmental health risk indicators reflecting potential risk to health, which provide another context for reviewing the effectiveness of interventions. All of these monitor changes in the health status of a population, often quite bluntly, over a period of time, and enable us to target specific areas to see if we have made an impact on morbidity.

However, the NHS exists in a cash-limited environment with well-rehearsed pressures on the available financial resources. In the past we were content with the concept of the health care professionals in the system using the resources available in the best interests of the individual. The NHS Executive's definition of health outcomes moved the goalposts quite subtly, by seeking the greatest improvement with the resources available of the physical and mental health of people in England and Wales. Their definition implies that those responsible for committing resources for the treatment and care of individuals should also be aware of the wider population and consider whether the health outcome for an individual is consistent with the greatest improvement to the population as a whole.

Historically, problems of both inequality of access and inequality of treatment have prevented some people receiving appropriate treatment. These problems remain today. The image of the NHS's universality is further undermined by the language it uses. NHS-speak is peppered with terms such as 'targeting' and 'eligibility criteria' which in themselves contradict any notion of availability for all . Expressions such as 'assessed health need' and 'clinical effectiveness' hint at the obstacles which need to be overcome. The continued confidentiality of clinical audit and the lack of freely available information about outcomes contributes to our uneasy awareness that the service system, in reality, is neither as systematic nor as effective as we would desire.

The government should publicly accept that this gives *de facto* recognition to the fact that the NHS is not, and probably has never been, the comprehensive universal service, free at the point of delivery, which it aspired to be.

For those who understand health care systems, none of this is either new or surprising. The definition of health outcomes by the NHS Executive reflects the aims of health care systems throughout the developed world, all of which face the same dilemma as we do in Britain. It may well be that we can take some comfort from just how cost-effective we have been with such a relatively small percentage of our national resources dedicated to health care. Where perhaps we do have a problem now is in recognising, and in conducting a debate about the fact that there will inevitably be an NHS which treats some people but, for the greater public good, declines to treat others. This problem has been exacerbated by the political importance of the NHS and the constant need of the main political parties to assert their commitment to the original principles of the service.

The effect of the continuing saga of NHS reforms of the

1990s has been to reposition the role of central government in this debate. Ever since Margaret Thatcher was given a hard time over the fate of a child in Birmingham, the aim of government has been to protect politicians from ever having to undergo a similar ordeal in the House of Commons. The devolution of resource and decision making in the NHS has now resulted in the situation where the NHS can be best understood by the following insurance analogy: central government is the principal insurer; health authorities and GP commissioners are the principal insurer's main agents; GPs, health trusts, other health professions, the private, voluntary and charitable sector are the health care providers or suppliers; and the people of Britain are the insured.

This chapter concentrates on the role of the insurers and the insured. It will not separately examine the roles of the health providers.

Central government – the principal insurer

Whatever they may really have believed, the previous governments of Mrs Thatcher and Mr Major publicly committed themselves to an NHS which was comprehensive and universal and free at the point of delivery.[27] Cynics would say that, having shot the albatross, the Conservative administration then hung it firmly around the neck of the next government, which would have had enough ideological trouble deviating from those principles, even without its newly acquired avian necklace.

The new government, led by Tony Blair, within a month

of taking office also committed itself to securing the delivery of equal access to health services for all the population on the basis of clinical need.[28] Thus, in the public's perception, the principal insurer has written a policy which still commits it to the tenets of comprehensiveness, universality and free service at the point of delivery. To move publicly and unilaterally away from these principles would require either a very brave government, or one which was certain it could bring with it a consensus of cross-party political views and national opinion following an open and informed debate. There have been few signs to date that central government is prepared to have this national debate.

Even if government did sponsor such a debate and was prepared, for instance, to consider introducing a hypothecated tax to fund the NHS, and to write the NHS insurance policy for its individual citizens, it is highly unlikely that the costs of administering the resulting system would actually decrease. The costs of processing claims and resolving disputes about the terms of the policy would be high.

The reality is clearly that central government, as the principal insurer, has developed alternative approaches to handling the conflict between its public commitment to the NHS and deliverable options to end users. They are:

- A system which transfers some costs directly to the consumers through prescription charges and fees for dental and ophthalmic services, and makes the cost of social care the responsibility of local authorities.
- An annual debate between the government as the

principal insurer, and the Department of Health as its head office, about the balance to be struck between the health care needs of people as policy holders, and the amount they are prepared to pay as a premium for health cover through taxes. Overall, this has resulted in a steady increase in the allocation of resources to the Department of Health for health care purposes. Unfortunately, this increase has not kept pace with the population's growing demand for health care, or with the rise of costs born of the system's increasing complexity and capacity to intervene.

- A system which delegates responsibility for decisions on rationing and priority setting to health authorities and GP commissioners (fundholders and locality commissioning groups) by:
  a. Reinforcing the role of GPs as the gateway to the NHS by offering them the opportunity to be not only providers but also purchasers of the health care services (as fundholders).
  b. Giving health authorities the responsibility for developing the insurance policy for the population in a particular area, based on a sound assessment - exercised in conjunction with GP commissioners – of the health care needs of the people in that area.
- A system of guidelines as to the quality of services which must be provided, and some outer limits (such as the stipulation that waiting lists must not exceed eighteen months) through mechanisms such as the Patient's Charter, and by establishing performance management and accountability arrangements. These link the Secretary

of State to Health Authorities and GP fundholders through the Chief Executive of the NHS Executive and the Regional Offices of the NHS Executive.

- A framework which:
  a. Gives support and encouragement to the development of clinical effectiveness.
  b. Gives support and encouragement to the audit of outcomes of treatment and care.
  c. Introduces the concept of eligibility criteria to the NHS in defined circumstances.

The Department of Health has also been careful to ensure that health authorities, in interpreting the national insurance policy, do not see it as excluding completely any particular types or forms of treatment or any particular people from access to that treatment. The central message has been that you may limit access to the system but never say that any individual is excluded from access to it. The central message has also, up to now, singularly failed to emphasise the responsibility of individuals as citizens as distinct from their rights. This may change with the change in government.

The principal insurer is responsible for evaluating health outcomes across the whole population which it insures. It has, with some hesitancy, introduced the concept of a 'health' service as distinct from a 'sickness' service through the Health of the Nation programme, and supported the role of Directors of Public Health in establishing a system of assessing the health care needs of local populations. The present government has strongly reinforced this role through the appointment of a minister with direct responsibility for public health issues. This provides an opportunity, at both national and local level, to reinforce the major contribution of organisations outside the NHS to the requirements of the public's health. It is less clear whether it also signals a step away from the sickness service and a step towards improving health outcomes (as desired by the NHS Executive).

Whether these policy commitments will enable the principle insurer to handle the conflict of interest between its health objectives and its financial objectives remains to be seen. Historically, as a monopoly insurer without competition, health outcomes have been less important to government than costs and volumes. Indeed, it is the pressure from the Treasury to demonstrate value for money and improved efficiency which has led to the focus on volume and efficiency as distinct from health outcomes.

Summary: the principal insurer

The principal insurer has:

- declined to determine what the insurance policy should cover
- declined to exclude any individual from cover
- thereby opted out of managing demand for health care
- delegated responsibility for the development of the group insurance cover to health authorities and, therefore, passed the dilemma on to them and to GP commissioners to work out with the health care providers and local people
- placed less emphasis to date on health improvement and health outcomes – despite the existence of the Health of the Nation Strategy, which requires long-term planning

and commitment – than on sickness services which are relatively short term in impact but respond to immediate issues of high public profile
- established a relatively effective system for maintaining central control and influence over their main agents – health authorities and GP commissioners.

Health authorities and GP commissioners – the principal insurer's main agents

Health authorities and GP commissioners have therefore, for both political and practical reasons, been delegated the task of developing the 'group insurance' policies covering their local populations. A whole range of contract policies has been developed, covering every aspect of health care from basic community services through to sophisticated specialist services. There has also been progress in the development of joint contracts with local authorities, covering both health and social care. Like commercial insurance policies these 'group insurance' policies seek to cover the main risks of ill health faced by the local population through the purchase of sickness services. Only a small percentage of the total resources has been devoted to prevention.

The response of health authorities and GP fundholders to the pressure on resources can be categorised according to whether they are acting on the supply side of the equation – via the efficiency and effectiveness of the providers; or on the demand side- through limiting the range of services or treatments covered by the 'group insurance' policy.

The issue of health outcomes can arise on both sides of this equation. Inevitably, in a situation in which resources are growing more slowly than the assessed health need, failure to make sufficiently rapid progress on the supply side leads to a reduction in the range of services which health authorities and GP commissioners can purchase through the 'group insurance' policy. It leads, in other words, to restrictions on the demand side.

Given the political and practical constraints which have prevented the principal insurer from more closely defining the NHS insurance policy, and given the desire to delegate responsibility to health authorities and GP commissioners, we might expect these bodies to have already assumed the main role in evaluating the effect of their commissioning policies on health outcomes. It is perhaps not surprising that progress in this has been variable, particularly given the plurality of commissioning bodies, the inherently different populations they serve, the differing provision for health and social care services already in place, and the very fact that they work in a bureaucratic system. It is perhaps worth examining four specific areas more closely: on the supply side of the equation – improved efficiencies and rationalisation; on the demand side of the equation – criteria for entry to treatment and care and criteria for exit from treatment and care.

1. Improved efficiency

To market-oriented health reformers of the late 1980s, it seemed self-evident that if even some of what was being practised in the name of treatment actually improved health, then greater efficiency in its provision would lead to an overall incremental improvement in the population's health. Although this statement may, to some, appear as naïve as Nye Bevan's idea that the NHS could ultimately end all illness, it held perhaps more than a grain of truth. There was little doubt that local NHS management often managed in name only, that hospitals were institutions which followed the whims of their medical consultant staff and that GPs were wholly unpredictable, unaccountable wildcards on the peripheries of the NHS.

Although some of the improved efficiency of providers in the 1990s may well have been because of better counting, overall the NHS is now securing more health care per pound than prior to 1990. Since the principal insurer has failed to clarify the contents of the insurance policy, it is questionable whether we are achieving the correct health outcomes from this improved efficiency. Very few health authorities have been brave enough to put more detailed clauses in the policy, and those that have done so have often found themselves exposed. GP direct purchasing has certainly moved participating GPs from the nether regions of the NHS closer to the centre of decision-making. Whether or not, after taking their management costs into account, they have been able to derive more health care from each NHS pound than any other purchaser, is still unknown. They have, however, had a questionable influence on overall outcomes. Most GP purchasers, whether they are GP fundholders or GP total purchasers, have shown great reluctance to take the responsibility for defining more narrowly the NHS insurance policy. Most would wish to leave that task either to their health authority or to national government.

The search for improved efficiency does, however, have its downsides. A holistic view of health outcomes is required in health and social care. Yet, the search for efficiency on the supply side has been applied to individual parts of the system, as opposed to the system as a whole. The result is that the search for improved efficiency has been accompanied by accusations of rising costs incurred when shifting between providers and poor quality of service for patients.

2. Rationalisation

Ultimately, the search for improved efficiency, at least in acute hospital services, has translated itself into the need for rationalisation of services onto fewer sites. This is in order to achieve reductions in overhead costs and improvements in the quality of service, consistent with new arrangements for medical staffing and the development of sub-specialty interests. Improving efficiency through rationalisation has, however, been a slow process owing to its unpopularity with local people, the introduction of new processes for handling capital investment and the lack of publicly available capital. These protracted processes have absorbed management energy and locked health authorities and Trusts into inefficient service provision, thereby reducing the quantity and the quality of service.

3. Criteria for entry to treatment and care

On the demand side, NHS activity is founded on the principle that GPs should act as the gateway to treatment and care. While this model is at best only a partial description of the health care system – there are a number of other ways of entering the system (such as through the Accident and Emergency wards) which bypass the GP – it has largely stood the test of time. It has been the foundation for the development of GP fundholding and other forms of GP-led commissioning. These have sought to link the GP's role in determining access to hospital and community health services with the financial responsibility for those decisions.

Although the language used in the health care system is somewhat different from that used in social services departments, the effect is often much the same. As the gap between people's needs and the resources available to meet those needs increases, and as ability to bridge that gap through further efficiency measures decreases, so eligibility criteria for access to care are raised. In the health care system, health authorities have sought to limit the cover provided by the 'group insurance' policy in two ways, both of which have their own repercussions:

i. Exclusions from contracts

While most health authorities have been careful to allow an 'appeal mechanism' in accordance with the central government requirements outlined above, there has been an increased tendency to identify clinical procedures and treatments which will be excluded from contracts. Exclusions, in terms of both treatments and prescription of medicines, are increasingly based around clinical effectiveness programmes and the identification of those procedures and treatments which are deemed to be clinically ineffective. This raises two questions: the first concerns the reliability of the evidence on which these decisions are based, the second the lack of a uniform approach throughout the NHS with differential effects on people as policy holders.

ii. Targeting

Targeting is the practice of identifying and targeting patients or groups of patients on the basis of assessed need. In terms of maximising health improvement from the resources available, and of taking steps to reach Health of the Nation targets, this approach seems thoroughly appropriate. It is, however, a system of selection – albeit one based on the assessed health needs of patients – which enables the prioritisation of limited resources. It is, in other words, a system of rationing access to health care. In reality the process has only just begun and has yet to seriously challenge the so-called inverse care law.

Currently the system operates on the assumption that individuals have the right to choose to attend the A&E department for a 'primary care' procedure, even though their GP receives a payment on their behalf in respect of such procedures. It is also frequently assumed that individuals have the right to another hospital out-patient appointment if they fail to attend the first. The system justifies this on a number of grounds:

- the concept of customer choice
- intra-system rivalry and lack of confidence, i.e. 'we can do the job better', 'it is impossible to get an appointment to see your GP', 'we are the provider of last resort'
- a justifiable desire not to victimise people with genuine difficulties

- the fact that it is often simpler to provide people with a service than to explain why it is not going to be provided
- the absence of a system for knowing if a patient arriving in, for instance, the A&E department, has or has not tried to contact their GP, or has already received telephone advice by the GP's out-of-hours service, rejected that advice and decided to go to the A&E instead.

Arguably, there is room for more debate about the responsibilities versus the rights of group policy holders. This debate may be particularly important in circumstances in which the actions of individuals deprive others of access to service. This, however, raises larger underlying questions about the criteria for entrance to treatment and care, which require a much more profound public debate, one which could possibly be sponsored by health authorities.

Such a debate needs to examine the appropriateness of commencing treatment in certain complex circumstances. The National Confidential Enquiry into Perioperative Deaths (NCEPOD) has, for instance, again drawn attention to the need for surgeons to consider and involve other specialists in decisions about the appropriateness of major surgical intervention on elderly people admitted as emergencies.[29] Audit evidence suggests poor health outcomes are the results of under-considered decisions. Similar difficult decisions have to be taken in respect of some types of cancer treatment. How does the clinician handle the expectations of patients and their relatives, along with their own feelings of inadequacy in such situations? The concept of multi-disciplinary assessment is much less advanced in acute situations than in the treatment of the mentally ill, and the system as a whole is programmed to intervention, rather than to reflection. The drive for efficiency, and the need for surgeons to get 'hands on' experience, can exacerbate this problem.

There is also a further dilemma surrounding the issue of compliance. We need to ask whether it is reasonable for people who, by their own actions and 'inactions', have contributed to their own poor health outcome, even after receiving appropriate specialist intervention, to continue to receive access to services at the expense of others.

4. The criteria for exit from treatment and care

This is another area which raises significant moral and ethical dilemmas, both for people in the health care system and for patients and relatives. The problem arises from the increased range of clinical interventions that are now possible, at increasingly high cost, particularly in specialist areas. The problem is where should treatment end, and where should intervention be replaced instead by maintenance or palliative care?

There are several dimensions to this dilemma. Patients are already frequently receiving treatment, and there are ethical and practical difficulties associated with discontinuing one treatment or moving patients to alternative and more appropriate forms of treatment. Also, since there is no insurance policy in place, there is no direct or external pressure on individuals to make a decision about the appropriate use of their own resources. This means that some of the tension is transferred to the relationship between patients and the clinical team caring for them. The clinician is faced with the problem of prioritising the clinical needs of the patient in accordance with the resources to which he or she has access in the system. Given the limitations on the total resources in the system, continued use by one patient often denies access to the service by others, who may have greater clinical requirements (and better health outcomes). Patients and their relatives can experience this tension as pressure, for example, to accept discharge or transfer to alternative forms of care. In a direct insurance-based system, some of this tension is diffused away from the clinical team to the relationship between individuals and their insurers.

As the new role for health authorities and GP fundholders as commissioners becomes better known, and as constraints are increasingly placed on clinicians, so there is also a steadily growing awareness of the role of the health authority and of the GP commissioner as the local insurer. Patients who feel that their needs are not being met are now being advised by health care providers and Community Health Councils (CHCs) to take up the issue with their health authority. A few patients are resorting to the Courts.

Summary: the principal insurer's main agents

The principal insurer's main agents have:
- made slow and variable progress in all areas
- improved supply-side efficiency
- begun to rationalise provider sites
- started to constrain the demand side
- still to grapple with cessation of treatment issues.

People in Britain – the insured

The effect on patients of the NHS framework set by the government and by health authorities and GP commissioners is by no means uniform across the country. People living in one health authority area will find that their 'group insurance' policy provides different cover from those registered with GP fundholders in their own area and from those living in other health authority areas. Sometimes variations will arise from genuine differences in the assessed health needs of local people. Sometimes they will result from the historical disposition of services in the area and at other times they are the results of different professional judgments or different routes into the health and social care system.

Despite these differences, there is a degree of shared experience by people using the NHS, resulting from the issues already outlined, and from social and technical change. Given the depth of some of the financial challenges facing the NHS, their impact on patients is likely to increase dramatically in the next few years. Four identified trends affecting individual patients as participants of a health authority negotiated 'group insurance' policy are:

i.   the transfer of responsibility for personal health back to the individual
ii. a continued reduction in the range of services available
iii. greater involvement of individuals, as local citizens, in identifying what should be included or excluded from their 'group insurance' policies
iv. the development of alliances between patients and

providers.

Let us look at each in turn.

1. The transfer of responsibility for personal health back to the individual

This trend is clearly discernible in a number of routine and everyday events. The move from in-patient to day-patient surgery transfers responsibility to the individual for determining whether their post-operative condition is satisfactory or unsatisfactory, and for arranging their domestic affairs appropriately. In fields such as diabetes and asthma, much greater emphasis has been placed on enabling people to cope with their condition, on giving them support and managing acute episodes in the community. Children are being taught from a very early age how to manage their own condition so they can maintain a normal lifestyle and avoid dependency on professional health care services. Similarly, health promotion aims to encourage people to make appropriate decisions about their health and lifestyle for themselves. A variety of arrangements have been put in place to enable people to access advice, both on general matters (through help lines) and on specific questions (through mechanisms such as telephone advice from GPs).

This approach is likely to be driven by the pressure of scarce resources and, given the right support, combined with systematic thought, can be taken much further. For example, the role of the community pharmacist is already being expanded, and can be developed more. Similarly, once ambulance services have responded to calls and evaluated the situation, and where the paramedic's assessment suggests a patient's condition does not warrant the use of an emergency response, they could decline to take patients on to hospital. Also, further thought and effort can be given to the interventions necessary to assist people who find it difficult to comply with treatment programmes, and who therefore repeatedly use general practice and hospital services.

We need to define the limits of this process quite clearly. Do we say to each smoker who has a coronary artery bypass graft that, if they continue to smoke and clog up their coronary arteries, they will be excluded from the insurance policy? Yet, even if there was local or national agreement to this, how would it fit with the training of health care professionals which advocates using their skills to help those they perceive to be in need? The indications from the furore surrounding those who have previously taken this kind of stance in public would suggest that we are not yet ready for such a step. Yet in reality, as most who work in the health service know, these decisions have already been made covertly.

The other side of this coin is that, if we are going to shift responsibility back to patients, they will rightly insist on having all the related facts available. We must not underestimate the difficulty of such a task, for it may well be that, once we have actually quantified the cost of the task versus the potential savings, we may decide it is not good value for money. Systematic strategic thinking on the part of the public service sector as a whole, rather than just the NHS, would enable people to take more responsibility for themselves, without recourse to financial penalty thresholds such as paying to visit GPs.

2. A continued reduction in the range of services available

Health authorities have been systematically reviewing the range of services available on the NHS and reducing it. Typically, the process began in peripheral areas such as tattoo removal and other minor cosmetic surgery. The range of items being excluded is extending significantly on the back of a growing emphasis on evidence-based medicine, and in response to financial pressures on the health authorities. This has led to variations between health authorities which look likely to remain. Having originated in the field of surgical procedures, the movement will extend to medical procedures. Here the evidence of effectiveness is more difficult to assess, but there are significant variations both in the referral patterns of GPs and in the response of hospitals to those referrals. These types of initiatives are likely to result either in a tighter definition of the clinical circumstances in which patients are deemed eligible for access to investigation, drugs and treatment, and/or in raising the threshold at which patients gain access to services. The overall effect is to narrow the cover provided by the 'group insurance' policy.

3. Greater involvement of individuals, as citizens, in setting priorities

As local authorities and GP commissioners become responsible for establishing priorities for services within the 'group insurance' policy, and as the pressure on resources grows, so the need to involve people in decisions as to which services are covered by the insurance policy also increases. Here the trade-off between the needs of the individual and the health of the population as a whole is at its most evident. If health authorities and GP commissioners are to be involved in identifying the criteria for entry to and exit from treatment, then they must share the task with local people and seek their input on the dilemmas discussed.

The majority of consultation undertaken to date has been about the rationalisation of service. It has scarcely touched the major moral and ethical decisions, which have principally been taken by clinicians, but which have an important bearing on resource utilisation in the NHS. In some circumstances – where a very small number of patients with severe and complex conditions are costing the service upwards of £500,000, or where a larger number of patients with growing clinical complications require increased clinical input and expenditure for diminishing health benefit – there may be a point at which the health needs of the population as a whole become greater than the needs and considerations of the individual. If so, how is this point to be identified, and how should the health authority facilitate discussion between local citizens and local clinicians, in order to promote an understanding of the issues and to reach some consensus on the road forward? However imperfect, and by whatever variety of methodologies, in future health authorities will make a greater effort to open up these issues to public debate and scrutiny, with all the personal, emotional and ethical dimensions that this will engender.

4. Development of alliances between patients and providers

Within any insurance-based system, even one as loosely defined as the NHS, there is always a debate between the policy holder and the insurance company as to the interpretation of the cover provided. The commissioners of health care (whether health authority, GP or central government) can expect to be lobbied both by individuals and by combined groups of patient provider and voluntary or charitable interests, on both the interpretation of the 'group insurance' policy cover, and on the range of treatments to be included in the NHS.

In conclusion, the NHS does not offer standard universal comprehensive sickness insurance to British citizens and the central government has recognised that it cannot, and should not, determine the content of the NHS insurance policy. The responsibility for determining the content of the service – what we have called the 'group insurance' policy – has fallen to health authorities and GP commissioners (GP fundholders). Central government has set out the general standards which should be met and the framework for the policy, and has given guidance on health care priorities. But responsibility for assessing local health care needs and for determining how resources should be allocated in order to meet those needs within the central policy framework, has also been delegated to health authorities and GP commissioners.

Since the resources available to them have not increased at the same rate as the desire to promote good health and the ability to treat patients, there has been, and will remain, pressure in the system for greater efficiency and assessment of relative health care need.

The parallel developments of clinical audit and evidence-based medicine have enhanced the ability of the NHS to consider and compare health outcomes with specific interventions. The combination of these factors is leading to a narrower definition of the cover provided under the 'group insurance' policy and to the transfer of some responsibilities and costs to the individuals covered by that policy. This trend can be expected to continue, allowing for geographical variations according to individual health authorities and GP commissioners.

Providers of health care can expect to be involved in discussions about the health outcomes they expect to achieve regarding proposed interventions, both prior to commencing, and during the course of treatment. In turn, local people, as 'group insurance' policy holders, can expect to become more involved, as local citizens, in the debates about effective health outcomes, and about moral and ethical issues regarding the interests of the individual versus those of the population group. In the future, the cover provided by the 'group insurance' policy is, however, likely to steadily reduce.

4. Shifting the Boundaries: Partnerships in Total Health Care

John Richards and Tony Shaw[10]

This chapter examines some of the current dilemmas of the British health care market and will consider various options 'beyond the NHS reforms' for reconciling needs and demands with the resources available. We will look at how these options are being carried out at present through locality commissioning in Southampton,[31] identifying the advantages of this approach and some of the potential pitfalls. Moving beyond the present idea of the 'purchaser/provider split' and building on the success of 'total purchasing',[32] we will go on to speculate on the more radical changes which may evolve, eventually leading to the integration of the provision of health care and perhaps borrowing some techniques and systems of managed care from America.[33]

It is now seven years since the introduction of the NHS reforms which established an 'internal market' aimed at delivering better value for money by introducing competition between providers. Now is a good time to take stock of what has happened, particularly since the new government is committed to evolutionary change.

The policy makers' expectation that competition between providers would increase efficiency has not, on the whole, been fulfilled. In practice, with the exception of London and Birmingham, there is little choice of providers for the majority of health care procedures (beyond the common elective procedures, which account for about 20 per cent of total expenditure). Economists agree that one of the essential conditions for efficient competition is that purchasers have 'perfect information'.[34] Experience has shown this is no more than a pious hope, and the Trust regime that was implemented has arguably engendered greater secrecy. It is now harder for purchasers to look at the figures behind the offered 'price' in order to understand providers' costing structures and manpower plans and judge the prices they are paying compared to others.

Fundholders have played the competitive market more successfully and have secured shorter waiting lists and sometimes preferential prices by threatening to move their business elsewhere and playing one provider off against another. Little is known, however, about the value for money they have achieved.[35] There have also been suggestions that fundholders have had more than their fair share of purchasing power, owing to the inadequate systems which set fundholder budgets.[36] Faced with increasing pressure on emergency and urgent services and reluctant to re-deploy resources solely from the 'non-fundholding' elements of their allocations, many health authorities during 1996–97 sought to redress the balance.[37] In Southampton, for example, analysis indicated that fundholders may have been over-generously funded to the tune of nearly £1 million (out of a total of around £35 million) and so budgets for 1997–98 were then reduced by half.

Of course, there are examples of purchasers using the leverage of competition to deliver better value for money, particularly through the market testing of clinical services. In Southampton, both learning disabilities and mental health services have changed in this way, but the process is highly resource intensive and often damages valuable local relationships. Such changes are worthwhile only when there appears to be no other way to deliver the necessary improvements in the quality of services.

In the general absence of competition, some commentators have promoted the concept of 'contestability' of provider prices.[38] As we will argue later, other factors have conspired to weaken the influence of purchasers over providers' behaviour and costs. Principally, provider costs (especially in acute care) have been driven by, and are even at the mercy of, rising demands. Purchasers have been left with the choice of either meeting the costs by diverting resources away from other priorities or negotiating with providers to limit their expenditure to keep costs down. On the whole, this is having less and less success and the result is that by the end of 1996–97 either purchaser or provider deficits are estimated to reach over £300 million nationwide. This chapter argues that a fresh approach to the problem is now needed.

The present dilemmas, though they were probably not the direct result of the reforms, have been exacerbated by them. They are the fundamental dilemmas of rationing faced by all health care systems which operate within financial constraints and rapidly increasing demand. The 1990 reforms forced these hard choices into the forefront and many commentators remain sceptical as to how genuinely open the subsequent priority-setting efforts of health authorities have been.[39]

We do not claim that the approaches promoted in this chapter are the only solution. They are simply a response to the dilemmas experienced within the present system. We assume that the founding principles of the NHS – a system which seeks to be comprehensive, based on equal access for equal need, largely free at the point of delivery and funded from general taxation – are still in keeping with the government's aims.

Similarly, we assume there may be little political desire to redefine the scope of what the NHS offers or to ration treatments at a national level, and that rationing or 'priority setting' will continue to be a local activity. We suggest that doctors and other practitioners should have a greater say in these kinds of decisions, particularly in regard to the interface between primary and secondary care. In the present environment, creative solutions are most likely to emerge from the kind of local initiatives being pursued in Southampton and elsewhere.

The real benefit of the reforms, possibly one unforeseen by the policy makers, has been the empowerment and mobilisation of primary care. The NHS's emphasis on primary care and the present enthusiasm among politicians and academics for locality commissioning and collaboration are to be welcomed. The danger is that their enthusiasm is only temporary and could easily evaporate.

As practitioners in the field, we are committed to an approach which centres on primary care, as we believe this is fundamentally right. The public believes that decisions about priorities should principally lie with the clinicians.[40] As the basic problem of managing demand occurs when deciding where to refer patients who require both primary and secondary care, primary care doctors have a leading role to play in taking these decisions. Locality commissioning should therefore be seen as a means of enabling them to make these choices more effectively.

Nevertheless, we are only too aware that our commitment to locality commissioning is largely an act of faith based on an approach which seems logical; there is little, if any, evidence that it has been fully implemented anywhere in the form which we propose, let alone that it works.[41] We are therefore determined to undertake a robust evaluation of the initiative as we proceed.

An additional theme which we will also discuss, and one which underlies our long-term vision, is the need to find better incentives, away from activity-based 'efficiency' measures which may promote overtreatment (especially in acute hospital care) and more in line with the systems which reward providers who maximise health gain (reduction in mortality or improvement in quality of life) within available resources.

Let us look at some examples. Southampton and South West Hampshire health authority is fairly typical, spending each year around £300 million commissioning health care for a population of over half a million people. The population, demographically speaking, is about average for the country and is relatively healthy and affluent, although there are significant pockets of deprivation. Within the authority's geographical boundaries is a major teaching hospital Trust which receives some £70 million out of a total annual expenditure on acute services of around £110 million. The authority is still below its 'target' allocation under the equity formula,[42] is well served in terms of primary care provision and has a strong history of collaborative strategic and practical work with social services and other partner agencies.

In 1997, the key issues facing the authority are:

- great financial pressure on its main acute service provider (Southampton University Hospitals Trust) which as a result is operationally limited
- the natural inflationary pressures of teaching hospitals (the need to be practising at the leading edge of medicine)
- the relatively easier access to high-cost interventions for the local population has created the potential for inappropriate or at least unaffordable levels of treatment
- the rising morbidity and exceptional underinvestment in mental health services of the city
- the low morale among many clinicians, nurses, GPs and managers.

A wider analysis suggests that the ability of purchasers (especially health authorities) to instigate change through contracting has been fairly limited, especially with regard to securing disinvestment and redeployment within or between providers to meet strategic priorities.[43] Perhaps the monopoly power of acute providers was inadvertently strengthened by the creation of Trusts – certainly their sense of corporate unity and cohesiveness has a potential downside when it comes to collaborative work with others in the wider interest of the population.

There is a serious dissonance between provider and purchaser planning systems, which seem to be operating in parallel universes. The following comparison illustrates their different mind sets:

Provider or Trust business strategy	Purchaser strategy
maximise business, market share, size	maximise population health
money should follow work	money should follow priorities
pay for what you get	get what you pay for
meet and manage demands	identify needs and allocate resources
development	redeployment
compete for business	rationalise and collaborate
maximise income	optimise resource use
reduce costs (cost improvement)	value for money (efficiency gain)
best services	best affordable care
clinicians do their best for individual patients	greatest good for the population

From this list, it is clear that Trusts have been encouraged to undertake a form of business planning which, arguably, has placed too much emphasis on maximising their market share and expanding services to compete with others for business. Their strategies are founded on the dangerous assumption that there is plenty more business out there to be 'captured' and, of course, paid for. Consequently, too little emphasis has been placed on ensuring that strategic direction is in line with purchaser priorities and their ability to pay.

Understandably, Trusts are wary of collaborative strategic initiatives which may threaten their market share. Only the more strategically realistic among them seem to have seen the impossibility of continuing in this vein (given the limited resources and the political needs to 'manage' the market) and now look to other providers and primary care practitioners as potential partners.

Our local experience suggests that the climate is now right to start encouraging these alliances, but there are still many inhibitions to be overcome. The environment must be created within which these quite different business strategies can flourish. In particular, the incentives which are currently created by the efficiency index [44] – which rewards increased acute activity regardless of its appropriateness – need to be replaced with targets for effective use of resources in improving health.[45] The new government has pledged action in this area and it will be interesting to see what proposals are put forward.

Some commentators go further than this and argue that we need to rethink the organisations in order to match care pathways and become more integrated and allow primary care physicians, GPs, greater influence on what happens in hospitals.[46] This responds to a fundamental dilemma of the present British health care system – how to manage more efficiently the interface between primary and secondary (and secondary and tertiary) care, so that the demands made on the more specialised (hence expensive) resources are the most appropriate (clinically speaking) and the rest is managed within a properly resourced primary care setting.

A first step along this road is being enthusiastically pursued in Southampton in the form of locality commissioning. This means that, as soon as is practically possible, the total local NHS resource (starting with hospital and community health services and prescribing allocations, and eventually general medical services) will be delegated to local groups of GP practices which have come together in 'natural' but rational groupings to commission health care on behalf of their practice populations.

Localities were first identified in the health authority's Health Strategy to the Year 2000 in 1994 and, a year later, lead GPs, each representing a locality, were appointed on a sessional basis to serve on a Core Commissioning Board alongside the chief executive and three executive directors of the Authority. Each locality is given a budget to purchase health care for populations of between 70,000 and 120,000. Some services will still best be purchased at a practice level, others will require a district-wide, and a few a supra-district, approach. This will be decided by the localities themselves in conjunction with the health authority.

The initiative did not emerge suddenly as a 'shaft of light' in board discussions at the Authority, but evolved from a series of practical discussions between managers and GPs. It became clear that there was a growing consensus about the way forward and the time was right for positive action. We believe locality commissioning will work because we have already seen the results of local groups of GPs taking control over resources and achieving changes in the delivery of services in line with the health authority's overall health strategies and priorities.

The Total Purchasing Project in Romsey, for example, involves three practices covering a population of around 35,000. In managing a budget which includes emergencies, the Romsey GPs have tackled their top three priorities by reshaping maternity services, changing their mental health provider and implementing a community-based model of rehabilitation, which has revitalised the local community hospital in the process.

The Southampton East Multi-fund covers twelve practices with 76,000 patients and an annual budget of £16 million. In 1996–97, the Multi-fund established a community mental health team to work in harmony with the health authority's mental health strategy and begin the process of reshaping local acute services to be more responsive to local needs. Its stated priorities for 1997–98 include cardiac surgery protocols, improved ECG reporting, shorter waits for rheumatology, the use of protocols for referral for joint replacement, provision of gynaecology outreach services and an integrated back pain service.

In some areas of the district, where 'total purchasing' or 'multi-fund' arrangements already exist, we expect full locality commissioning to proceed in April 1999. In other areas, it will take a little longer. This is not an approach which is being forced upon GPs by the health authority, but one which has emerged from the success of existing arrangements which go part of the way, and is aimed at both parties now proceeding together in partnership. The management resources of the health authority will be reorganised to support these arrangements.

We expect locality commissioning to deliver purchasing which is more sensitive to local priorities but also provides arrangements to pool risk and minimise transaction costs. By creating a 'total' budgetary system, localities can strike an appropriate balance between elective and emergency priorities in a way that was difficult under the limitations of standard fundholding. Effective working relationships with providers of social care will also be important, especially in building on the success of pilot projects which have enabled practices to include care managers and access social services resources to provide more integrated community care.

Most importantly, we believe that localities represent the best hope of promoting clinical effectiveness in practice, by combining clinical and budgetary responsibilities with the flexibility to match the intervention chosen (including drug therapies) to the needs of each patient. We believe that localities will prove an effective vehicle for enabling providers of secondary care to change the services they provide so that they better meet the needs of their patients.

This is not to say the approach is without potential pitfalls. The following are among the most obvious:

- not all GPs are natural participants, and some will need considerable encouragement to see the benefits locality commissioning will bring to patients and themselves
- linked with this, there is a clear demand for adequate resourcing of locality management, including the time spent by GPs on commissioning as opposed to primary care provision, which must be reconciled with the continuing downward pressure on management costs
- there are obvious risks to financial control inherent in delegating resources in this way, as some health authorities have found to their cost, and careful work is required to develop further appropriate financial policies and performance management arrangements without stifling the localities
- considerable demands will be made on information

management and systems to meet the needs of localities and, although considerable investment has been possible through the fundholding initiative, a major challenge lies ahead

- the 'big picture' must be kept in focus – handling the major strategic issues and market instabilities. Health authorities are expected to 'hold the ring', but it is an ill-defined role and will call for a delicate balance to be maintained between local freedoms and strategic priorities.[47]

In many ways, however, locality commissioning may be only a step along the road towards a more radical future. Several commentators have compared 'total purchasing' to the Health care Maintenance Organisation (HMO) model of managed care in America and asked what other aspects of managed care might also be transferred to Britain.[48]

Our vision of a possible future includes four key elements:

1. Vertically or virtually integrated 'total health care' providers encompassing primary and secondary care, which evolve out of the present localities for commissioning.
2. Trusts redefined as managers of facilities and providers of highly specialised 'technical' clinical services.
3. Capitation-based payments from health authorities to the total health care providers based on agreed programmes of care.
4. Financial incentives for health gain.

Importantly, in view of the criticisms in this chapter of the current organisation of provision, we believe there is a need to 'break the link' between institutions (such as hospitals or Trusts) and the clinical teams who deliver services. Total health care providers could develop, which link the primary care physicians (GPs) and at least some of their secondary care colleagues (most obviously, general and geriatric physicians, paediatricians and gynaecologists). Robinson and Steiner anticipate the emergence of this sort of model in Britain and suggest that such 'tight' organisational forms seem to have the greatest impact on performance.

The secondary care clinicians could be either employed by the total health care provider itself (the vertically integrated model) or linked to it through contractual agreements but remain essentially self-employed (the virtually integrated model). These clinicians would gain access to hospital facilities, where appropriate, through agreed 'admitting rights'. In turn, the total health care provider would provide care for an enrolled, i.e. registered, population in return for a capitation-based payment (not unlike the locality budgets proposed). This care could be provided in a variety of settings (including hospitals) according to the appropriate clinical needs and the best use of resources. The capitation payments could be linked to specific integrated programmes of care (such as circulatory diseases, mental health, diabetes and so on), enabling the health authorities to set priorities between different health problems according to national and local policies, but allowing for the providers to retain the flexibility to determine when, where and how to intervene for their registered patients in order to deliver health gain.

There would be incentives within the system to encourage these behaviours and to invest in health promotion where it is cost-effective in achieving health gain. In America, for example, Kaiser Permanente, the foremost American managed care organisation, provides regularly updated health promotion literature to its enrolled population because it believes this is effective in reducing the demand for more costly interventions further down the line.[49]

In these new clinical partnerships for the provision of total health care, some of the age-old problems linked to the use of the health estate may also be solved. Trusts would essentially become facilities managers (like airports) and, with the tie between care and buildings loosened, the scope for rationalisation of the estate could be much greater.

Nevertheless, there may be a place for competition within such a model. It could be introduced at a number of levels:

- between Trusts to secure business from the admitting secondary care clinicians
- between the secondary care clinicians themselves to join total providers
- between total providers to attract practices of GPs to join them or, in a yet more radical form, to attract patients.

This last option, where the individual patient exercises choice to enroll in the best provider scheme, is not without potential problems, chief among which is equity. For such a model to function fairly, the two preconditions would be:

1. that a real choice exists for all individuals (including those who cannot afford to travel out of their immediate vicinity to receive care)
2. that consumers (patients) have access to meaningful information about the performance of alternative providers.

Neither of these preconditions would be easy to achieve, but safeguarding them may be an important function of health authorities in the future.

Alternatively, or as an interim step, the choice to affiliate with alternative providers could lie with GP practices, deciding on behalf of their patients. Again, adequate protection for the rights and interests of patients would need to be ensured.

This model has several features in common with the American HMO, except that here the insurer is the state. This is not to say that we are advocating every aspect of the American system, which we believe to be riddled with inefficiency and inequity in many respects. An attractive analogy was used by Professor Brad Kirkman-Liff from Arizona State University on a recent study tour to Britain.[50] He described the American system as a chaotic 'jungle', compared to the 'well-ordered garden' of the NHS. Nevertheless, with caution it may be possible and advantageous to transplant some specimen plants from that jungle into our garden.

We believe this model is consistent with the founding principles of the NHS as a publicly financed system. It leaves open the question of the 'ownership' of the provision of health care, which admittedly many see as a *sine qua non* of the NHS. It would be possible, in our model, for the ownership of the NHS estate either to remain in public hands or to be taken over by private investors. Clinicians could continue to be employed independently by Trusts or by Total Health care Providers, or they could be self-employed or even employed by health authorities. Similar options would exist for GPs and practice staff.

This may seem a long way from the present realities facing the NHS, but the move towards locality commissioning opens up some exciting possibilities. If we do decide to proceed in this direction, we will need the willing partnership of all the professionals and other stakeholders involved to make it work. Ways of facilitating their involvement should form the basis of any emerging national strategy for the NHS.

5: The Future of Mental Health in a Community Setting

Trevor Turner

A leading article in the *British Medical Journal* in 1990 opened with the sentence 'community care is not working'.[51] It then went on to analyse the reasons for this, looking at the paradoxes, uncertainties in definition and fragmented policies that provided the background to the community approach. And, in the public eye at least, the notion that community care has failed has become increasingly accepted as the decade has progressed. This pessimism reflects the increasing expectations placed on the health service in general, the rejection of the post-war liberalism that initiated the closedown of the traditional asylums, and a misunderstanding of the processes and practices of community care.

The switch from asylum-based care, which started in the late 1950s and flourished in the 1960s and 1970s, was generated by both technical and attitudinal changes. Most non-clinical commentators tend to gloss over the enormous impact of modern medications, while stressing the obvious failings of institutionalisation and segregation inherent in the large, isolated, Victorian mental hospitals. The demise of these hospitals was predicted in the famous 'Watertower' speech, made by the then Minister of Health, Enoch Powell, in 1961.[52] Deinstitutionalisation became the accepted approach throughout Europe and North America, driven by popular understanding of mental illness as outlined in the radical tracts of R.D.Laing, films such as *One Flew Over the Cuckoo's Nest* and a flourishing anti-psychiatry movement. Until the late 1970s, graphs illustrating the falling number of psychiatric beds in the health service, and the reduced use of detention under the terms of the Mental Health Act, were warmly received.[53]

At the same time, carefully conducted research using a random selection of patients (in hospitals or community treatment centres in crisis) also demonstrated the clear benefits of the move towards dedicated community teams.[54] These benefits were seen in patients' and families' preferences, decreases in apparent costs and reductions in the time spent in hospital over the course of an illness. By and large, surveys of patients cared for in community settings (which is to say, individuals living independently, with their families or in very small residential homes) reported an increase in patients' social contacts and a continuation in their psychiatric stability.[55] But from the 1980s onwards this trend of progressive improvement started to disintegrate. This was partly because of unfounded optimism as to the effectiveness of community care, and in particular the unavailability of the bridging funds required to set up and run community teams while maintaining hospital care. Rising unemployment and homelessness, the constant shortfalls in health and social service funding and an increasing public awareness of 'untoward incidents', added to the public's disillusion. In a series of powerful articles in the *Times*, the campaigning journalist Marjorie Wallace led the call for a re-evaluation of asylum closures.[56] The isolation and poverty of poorly supported patients (often chronic schizophrenics), living in grubby bed and breakfast accommodation, showed how vulnerable the sufferers of mental illness, and the mental illness services in general, were to broader economic and social changes.

There is a great deal that we can learn from the dilemmas

and arguments that resulted from this policy change. Although there had been some unrealistic projections as to the numbers of beds required, and little understanding as to what community work entailed, the traditional asylum setting was revealed as unnecessarily custodial and liable to abuse. Furthermore, the criticisms of diagnostic and therapeutic practices within psychiatry shook the profession out of a certain complacency. Improved training programmes, a renewed interest in psychopharmacological and brain metabolism research and the establishment of robust diagnostic criteria, demonstrated how unscientific were the traditional frameworks of psychotherapy and institutional rehabilitation.[57] Fresh air was let into the system.

Let us look at each of the dilemmas in turn.

Public disenchantment

Mental illness is still an area of considerable sensitivity even though the stigma has been substantially reduced over the past fifty years. Media coverage remains largely sensational, preferring the 'mad axeman' story to the quiet uninteresting lives of the majority of those with chronic mental disorder. Typical cartoons show, for example, a doctor and a patient in a bleak room, with the doctor saying 'now we are going to play a game called "Hunt the Bed"' or King Lear and the Fool, on the blasted heath, with the latter saying 'I knew they would put us out to care in the community, Lear'. In fact the phrase 'community care' has now come to signify irrationality and neglect.

The regular publication of outrages and 'untoward incidents', such as the 1994 Ritchie Report into the care of

Christopher Clunis (who stabbed a passer-by in a North London tube station, without provocation), do much to enhance public fear.[58] Naturally enough, the stigma also stretches to those who work in mental health whether they be nurses, doctors or care workers (note how common are statements such as 'you're the only sane psychiatrist I know'). In fact this stigma extends much more widely in day-to-day living than is generally recognised. For example, most psychiatric patients who have obtained work admit to not having told their employers of their illness history. Private hospital treatment plans almost always exclude mental illness, except in the very small print at the bottom. If you take out medical insurance for a holiday abroad and develop a mental illness, as opposed to say malaria, your bills will not be paid, although the former is often more disabling. As a result not only do individuals try to deny their own illness but families collude in covering it up, which leads to delays in treatment. The lack of any outward, visible sign of disorder means that patients are often regarded as not 'deserving'. And it is common for schizophrenics, though stable on medication, to be rejected, and disbelieved, as witnesses in court.

Defining community

The somewhat tautological definition of community care is 'care delivered in the community rather than in total institutions'. Thus it is not a form of treatment, such as analytical psychotherapy, nor even a coherent philosophy; if anything it is a sociological construction, based on the sense of normalising individuals' lives as much as possible despite their handicap or disability. There is little attempt to define the notion of community in most of the writing on community care for the mentally ill, and much of the research has taken place in relatively middle-class areas of North America and Australia. Thus the assumption that any community will be able to cope with this approach is not based on any research into more fragmented communities, such as the inner cities. The populations there are largely transient with substantial numbers of people unemployed or living in public housing. There are many single parent families and a limited number of individuals, particularly in the voluntary sector, who are able to offer support.

Furthermore, a wide range of provision is required within the context of 'community care', but it is difficult to justify highly professional support for what is a relatively mundane task in terms of continuing care. Patients tend to vary in their support needs, depending on the stages of their illness, and problems of personal isolation and the need for occupation are often particularly difficult to resolve. The shortage of housing and jobs further marginalises the disabled psychiatric patient, while the increased demand for services of all sorts dilutes the professional support which is available.

Carers

There has been considerable research on the role of carers, both in professional journals and by family support organisations such as the National Schizophrenia Fellowship (NSF).[59] One of the most recent reports has outlined the fact that many carers are female, older and experience violence intermittently as part of their caring role. They are often isolated, yet provide the backbone for much of what is done. Hence the tacit and ironic alternative definition of community care as the 'transfer of care to untrained staff'. In terms of professional carers, there is no such animal as a 'generic' community care worker. Carers come from a wide range of health backgrounds and are usually community psychiatric nurses, occupational therapists or psychologists, with social workers often attached to the care team.

Between them, these professionals and the carer (usually the mother) will be asked to look after individuals with changing needs depending on their illness status. Not only will the patient often have to trek from the community care office to the social work office to the benefit office (and as often as not to the housing office) in order to obtain what he or she needs, but there is frequently no clear definition as to what skills are required by the relevant professionals. Essentially the support involved is a mixture of friendship, counselling, practical advice (such as help in form-filling) and the provision of medication. There remains little outside recognition of the disparate nature of these tasks.

Mental Health Act

The current Mental Health Act (MHA) was passed in 1983, and outlines the procedures for treating patients against their will, as well as the various processes for protecting patient rights. It contains 149 paragraphs or 'sections', and the phrase 'requires treatment in hospital' is central to the definition of those requiring involuntary treatment. In other words, anyone who develops a serious mental illness, and about 12 per cent of all admissions to mental hospitals in Britain come under the terms of the MHA, has to be placed in hospital. Despite the emphasis on community care, and the constant focus on providing help outside institutions, hospitals continue to be an essential part of the provision of a comprehensive service.

There is no such thing as a community treatment order in England and Wales, although under section 41 of the MHA it is possible for a judge in a crown court to impose a 'restriction' order. This is a somewhat heavy-handed section – it normally requires patients to be treated in hospital for several years, sometimes longer, and then undergo a prolonged period of leave outside hospital under 'conditional discharge'. It also requires the patient to have committed an act so 'untoward' that he or she is deemed to pose a serious risk to the public. It is a classic case of shutting the stable door after the horse has bolted, and cannot help community teams prevent dangerous incidents, even if they suspect they may take place in the future. It is generally accepted that reform of the MHA is required, but it is difficult to make parliamentary time available. New Acts in this field generally get passed every twenty or thirty years. This century, for example, they were passed in 1930, 1959 and 1983, the Lunacy Act of 1890 having remained largely in force until 1959. So change is unlikely before the millennium.

Costs and resources

Government support for community care was, in part, based on the notion that it would be cheaper, given the fixed costs and large capital resources involved in maintaining traditional asylums. It was an obvious assumption that individuals living at home, possibly even working part-time, even if they did require some form of disability benefit, would not increase costs for the National Health Service. The rise in the Social Services budget over the last few years has been one natural outcome (among other processes) of the community care policy. But more sophisticated economic analyses have shown that community care is probably in the end no cheaper than asylum care.[60] Furthermore, sales of asylum land and property were undermined by the collapse in the housing market in the late 1980s, while the costs of looking after individuals in smaller, more home-like, units rose.

An important follow-up study, based on the closure of Friern Hospital in North London, followed eight annual cohorts of patients discharged until the hospital closed in 1993.[61] While the first four cohorts could be placed in relatively low support accommodation, the last four proved increasingly costly to house and care for. This is not surprising, since they were the most disabled and severely ill patients, which is why they were last to be discharged. The cost of caring for this group of patients in a community setting was much higher than keeping them in hospital, and the overall cost of both low and high dependency patients proved slightly higher than if they had continued to stay in hospital.

When one considers that mental health care has also lost out in terms of NHS funding by at least one per cent over the last five years, and that there has been increasing pressure from the prison services to take mentally-disordered offenders (with concomitant extra costs in finding expensive medium secure or high security places), it is clear that there are no obvious economic benefits from a community care approach. The introduction of General Practitioner (GP) fundholding has also placed further demands on mental health services to provide more support for those patients with less severe mental illness (the so-called 'walking worried'), because it is these rather than schizophrenics who fill GP surgeries.

The social/health crossover

Defining the boundaries between social service provision and NHS provision has never been easy. The increasingly complex needs of individuals with chronic mental health problems, or with the disabilities of old age, have highlighted this. An eighty-year-old lady, for example, who has suffered a stroke, has limited self-care abilities, symptoms of secondary depression, but fiercely insists on living independently, requires elements of both services. Generating joint resources in terms of eliding social service and health provision, has only recently come on to the political agenda. Although there has been some development of combined mental health and social work teams, the varying management structures, significantly different pay scales, and the distinct priorities of the two forms of service, tend to impair co-ordinated work. It is not surprising that such poor co-ordination is typically found in enquiries into 'untoward incidents', whereby information from one agency has not been passed on to the other, leading to delays in treatment and thus the patient becoming increasingly unwell.

In particular, there are certain perverse incentives built in to the funding arrangements for both agencies. All NHS provider units (that is to say, hospitals) define remunerable activity on the basis of admissions. This has traditionally been based on the Full Consultant Episode (FCE) which in itself has only an indirect relationship to the actual cost of a specific admission. Yet a mental health unit that avoids admissions is seen as not requiring remuneration, and is likely to suffer cuts in its budget. Likewise it is much cheaper for a social services department to admit people to hospital, and keep them there, rather than transfer them to the community where costs to their budget will be incurred.

From these core dilemmas it is possible to outline a number of significant pressures on the future prospects for community care in mental health. An underlying theme behind all these is the insidious demand, from various agencies, for the return of the traditional asylum or mental hospital. This is seen as a safe and humane option, largely because people have forgotten about the number of hospital inquiries held in the 1960s and 1970s, which revealed the incidence of abuse within such a closed system. In addition there is widespread acceptance of the rising demand for mental health services associated in general with an ageing population, the increasing awareness of symptoms and treatments and the trend towards the 'medicalisation' of social ills. Furthermore, the tendency of the acute hospital sector (medicine and surgery) to 'resource-raid' community mental health services is largely hidden from the general public, and is underestimated even by those working within the service.

Let us look at a number of the pressures which have arisen.

Public rejection

Negative attitudes to mental health problems have been inherent in the development of community care, and certainly preceded the rise of the asylum. In fact, the success of the asylum as a policy initiative for dealing with the increasingly visible numbers of mentally ill in an urban environment, was derived in part from its ability to segregate those deemed a threat to 'normal' society. In modern terms, the phenomenon of 'nimbyism' (not in my back yard) especially affects the location of, for example, after-care mental health hostels. A recent survey, by the patients' organisation MIND, found that two in three of its local area organisations had encountered opposition to mental health facilities in the past five years.[62] Fear was the main focus of concern, expressed as fear for children's safety, fear of violence and falling house prices in the surrounding area. There have even been reports of random attacks, usually by young people vandalising property or threatening staff and ex-patients, an attitude which substantiates the idea that community care really means treating 'other people, somewhere else'. Furthermore, the more difficult the potential client group is seen to be (for example, mentally disordered offenders, or those with drug or alcohol problems) the higher the level of local hostility.

The effect of this is twofold. Not only is it difficult to find residential places for those at most risk of relapse, thus increasing the pressure to keep such people in hospital, but hostels themselves become selective. In order to maintain their credibility within the local community, hostels carefully screen out individuals who might be seen as 'at risk', through formal and relatively lengthy assessment procedures. This selection of the most suitable residents is understandable, although it does seem that once residential projects have opened, whatever their clientele, local opposition usually fades very quickly. Nevertheless there is a 'stage army' of rejected patients, often those with more complex needs and illnesses, who tend to drift from hostel, to prison, to the street and back into hospital. Such individuals are typical of those at the centre of 'untoward incident' inquiries, but this fearful public response also creates pressures for readmission within the hospital system. Thus the more community placements there are in a given area, the more likely it is one will require additional acute beds for respite care, relapse care and to deal with this heightened sensitivity.

The community

There are considerable limits to a community's willingness to support individuals who are 'difficult to manage'. Although there may be sympathy among individuals, even communities with a strong and stable family base and a minimal transient population tend to reject those with aberrant behaviours. It is an established fact of social research since the 1930s, that patients with very complex needs, particularly those with schizophrenia, tend to drift to the inner cities. The very nature of their illnesses, for example paranoid delusions, tends to incorporate the local environment into the problem as perceived by the patient. Once recognised and stigmatised within the small town or local community, retreat to the anonymity of the inner city becomes something of a relief to the patient. Thus setting up successful community care facilities in suburban or rural areas can be relatively easy since, by definition, many of the more demanding patients will have left the area. Such facilities, or models of care (and much of the research into community care has been based in stable communities), should not be used as models for practice in more socially deprived areas.

It is interesting to note that in the past the establishment of a specified 'catchment area', for which a particular hospital is responsible, traditionally applied only to geriatric and psychiatric units. This was in order to protect hospitals from being 'dumped' with difficult patients with long term care needs. For example, the current costs of a placement in a medium secure unit are approximately £100,000 per annum. So in London, for instance, if only a few members of the transient population (there is a 30 per cent turnover in NHS surgery registrations in most of inner London) become unwell, end up in prison and require such care, the relevant health authority will find itself £200,000 or £300,000 a year in the red.[63] This is the equivalent of employing ten community psychiatric nurses. Given the rising tide of expectation as to levels of support required outside hospitals – such as daily visits or access to a day centre at evenings and weekends – the balance between acute care, respite care and after-care is constantly shifting.

Carer support

There have been increasing reports of 'burnout' among the families and professionals looking after those with chronic mental illness.[64] Accentuated by social stigma and deprivation, it is as often as not the chronicity of the disorder that causes most despair. Elderly parents find it more problematic to cope, and respite care resources (in order to give the carer a break or a holiday) are usually few and far between. There is also poor recruitment within mental health and social services, particularly in the poorer areas. But when agency staff are employed the quality of care is reduced and levels of violence increase on units where locum nursing staff are employed. Likewise, the very vulnerability of the clientele, who often rely on personal support and contact for many of their most basic needs, enhances the extent to which they are exploited. And the initiatives aimed at providing more active support are often confronted by fragmented funding arrangements.

This situation is worsened by the often bewildering variation in the agencies with whom a carer may have to negotiate. Housing departments are notoriously under pressure, while social services tend to be dominated by the needs of the elderly and child protection. Often it is the local policeman, or the local shopkeeper or just a concerned neighbour, who knows most about a vulnerable person's condition. Such *ad hoc* support is rarely coherent, and is easily exacerbated by the limited availability of the professional. Paying such volunteers usually requires creative accounting subterfuges.

Supervision demands

Although there is some evidence that the breakdowns in care highlighted by critical inquiry reports, and published in the media, have helped to secure additional community mental health funding, they have also created considerable pressures.[65] There have been growing demands for intervention by the courts and the legal system, leading to an increase in the number of psychiatric assessments before disposal and stern requests by judges or magistrates that prolonged admission and or supervision is adhered to by the mental health team. The hasty policy decision to introduce a 'Supervision Register', in the aftermath of the Christopher Clunis affair (1994), is an example of one such outcome.[66] Under this measure, which was introduced via an Executive Letter and had nothing to do with the MHA, all mental health units were told to draw up a list of individuals 'at risk' under various criteria. These included the risk of self-harm, the risk of hurting other people and the risk of self-neglect. No additional powers in terms of treatment or therapeutic activity, no additional resources and no specific benefit to the patient (apart from life-long stigmatisation) were included in this package. The core pressure was to increase the responsibility of the local mental health team for any breakdown in care, and to reduce the potential liability of central government, which actually provided the resources.

This measure was followed by the 'Supervised Discharge Order', under the terms of the Patients in the Community Act of 1996. This gave powers to the Responsible Medical Officer (RMO) to order a patient to live in a particular house or residence, to have access to that place of residence at any time and to 'convey' the patient to or from a hospital unit, if concerned about their mental health status. Again, there were no powers of treatment granted and the measure very much reflected fears about public order rather than a therapeutic concern for the well-being of vulnerable patients. It might be suggested that the whole notion of supervision in the community is in itself an oxymoron.

One reason for these measures is the marked shortage of medium secure beds, and the increasing pressures on the general hospitals, as well as the high security units, because of this. Such units are expensive, and community teams are often reluctant to accept those who are discharged from them because of the potential difficulties involved. There are known pressures within the prison system: reports indicate that 30–50 per cent of prisoners have significant mental health problems, and prison health care facilities are often variable in size and quality.[67]

Funding

Despite its definition as a 'priority' service, mental health care (and care of the elderly) is usually seen as a 'Cinderella' service. This reputation is reflected in the nature of the buildings in which such units are found (Victorian workhouses, the older wings of hospitals) and their limited resources in terms of revenue and capital. A particular problem is the difficulty relating outcomes to costs, in contrast to the ready packages available for 'cold' surgery or more defined medical procedures. Essentially the patient with mental illness will often require a commitment to longer-term funding, reducing the flexibility of resources in terms of strategic planning.

In addition the complex range of funding sources – which are increasingly short-term in order to meet political challenges – tends to inhibit strategic development. Typical examples are the London Initiative Zone funds (LIZ) and the Challenge Funds for various mental health initiatives.[68] These are especially vulnerable to temporary or political pressures, and are more often allocated to areas with good presentational skills rather than areas in greater need.

From the patient's point of view there are regular changes in their allowances, for example, the Disability Living Allowance (DLA), which mean that they have to make constant re-applications for continued funding, because of the squeeze on the Social Services budget. Rising government concern about the numbers claiming Invalidity Benefit has led to closer review of an individual's status, and a tendency to reject those without an obvious physical disability. At a broader level, the funding formulae for a given health area do not include a 'homelessness' factor, and underestimate capitation figures where immigrant groups and transiency are common.

The social/health divide

The pressure created by rising homelessness, shortfalls in funding and the lack of housing demonstrates the inadequacy of the co-ordination between government departments. This was highlighted in the 1994 Parliamentary Health Committee Report, 'Better off in the community?', but the issue still remains unaddressed and a source of increasingly bitter wrangling.[69] As a result it has become established practice for all participants in the community care game to attempt to shift responsibility, especially for the more costly, 'difficult to manage' clients. Admission criteria, changing definitions and Risk Assessment are the various tools of the trade.

This problem of defining responsibility was reflected in the introduction of the Care Programme Approach (CPA). Based on establishing a defined keyworker, assessment of need and regular monitoring of the action required, this approach has certainly developed an admirable model of good practice. However, lack of resources to meet the defined needs, the subsequent delay in discharging patients from hospital and remorseless demand for more meetings and more paperwork (hence its acronymic alternative, Continuous Paper Accumulation) have tended to clog up the system and enhance exasperation among care workers and families.

The most overt pressure, within the social/health interface, is suitable housing. Chronic mental illness can in part be defined as an inability to look after a normal domicile without support. Yet obtaining placements (especially in shortage areas, or where local tenants are hostile, or when an individual has already damaged his or her previous housing) can be impossible. Whereas the old asylum did, in management terms, combine the ability to treat, occupy and house the mentally ill, the relationship between Housing and Social Services departments in many boroughs is one of hostile mistrust. This has been enhanced by policy arrangements, such as the Homeless Mentally Ill initiative, whereby responsibility for differing elements in the package required contributions from the Housing Corporation, the Department of Health and local authorities. The very complexity of arrangements, at all levels of the system, is used in itself to deflect demand, which creates unfair pressures for those on the front-line.

The policy issues generated by these dilemmas and pressures need to embrace both an historical and a strategic view of provision for the mentally ill. Social stigma, community, professional roles, legislation, funding arrangements and government structures will all have an impact on development. It is also important to agree on a clear commitment to the philosophy of community care, based on the idea of 'normalisation' of those individuals marginalised by illness or disability. This is not an empty optimism, but will become more likely in the future through advances in modern drugs, reductions in the causes of illness and the simplification of arrangements in social organisations. Such a commitment will need clear and co-ordinated support in terms of presentation and funding. Reactive demands for a 'bricks and mortar' solution will continue to be made, just as they were being made even in the heyday of asylum provision, particularly when there was public outrage involving a mentally ill individual. Emphasising the benefits to society that accrue from a humane policy towards the mentally ill will have to be part of the project.

Stigma

The current in-built practices supporting stigma and 'nimbyism' will need to be sensitively addressed. There has been little direct confrontation, unlike the campaigns on behalf of other disenfranchised groups (for example, homosexuals or the elderly) to avoid antagonising potential allies. However, any statutory provision to prevent discrimination in employment will have to be balanced by an acceptance of short-term contracts or differentiated agreements on sick pay provision. Likewise, the development of a campaign along similar lines to the anti-racism campaign, would need to choose its words carefully. The term 'mentalism' has been used, but there is a tendency for such words to be quickly abused, while constant shifts in acceptable terminology (for example, the switch from 'mental handicap' to 'learning difficulties') avoid the issue. Better health education in schools, including an understanding of psychiatric disorder, as well as the portrayal of illnesses such as schizophrenia in popular TV series (for example, the character Joe in *Eastenders*) can only be evaluated over the long term. An understanding that such approaches may take several generations to achieve their full impact may diminish enthusiasm for funding in the short term.

Community

Developing research into the care of the severely mentally ill within more deprived settings is an obvious approach. Given the limited resources available, the acceptance of certain 'mini-institutions' as a historical half-way house between the relatively economical asylum and the costly individual home, has already become a feature in this area. Personal freedom and one's own style of living is seen as the essence of community care, but this does not preclude acceptance of some supervision and certain statutory requirements. Communities which agree to hostels for mentally disordered offenders, for example, could be rewarded in terms of local tax credits. An incentive to prevent unpopular or 'difficult' patients from moving on would need to be matched by resources that include a quotient for homelessness. Policies aimed at stabilising inner-city communities, in terms of local employment, school provision and the broader prevention of alcoholism and drug dependence, will need to be integrated with these provisions.

Professional roles: carers

Those looking after vulnerable people provide the backbone of community care, whether it is for the mentally ill, the elderly or children. Providing payments for members of the family, for example via the current Disability Living Allowance, always involves bureaucracy and regulations. Directing payments at 'wellness' rather than disability could involve patients accepting medication or other treatment programmes in order to qualify for such payments. The ability and responsibility to look after one's own money needs to be integrated within mechanisms such as medical sickness certificates, along similar lines to the schemes in parts of America. Likewise, those currently acting as community care workers may have to accept the evolution and eventual abolition of their traditional status. This will ruffle professional feathers, but there is no obvious reason why an individual capable of giving an injection should not be able to sign a mental health order, or obtain a bus pass or vice versa. New training programmes, new forms of qualification and inter-professional disputes over such developments, as well as over comparative pay scales, will have to be accepted in order to promote a longer-term view. Tax benefits for those involved in voluntary work will also have to be considered.

Legislation

New statutory powers and arrangements, under a revised Mental Health Act, will necessarily be controversial. The power to treat an individual against his or her will is based upon the acceptance of a right to care when patients are unable to judge correctly for themselves. However, the European Convention on Human Rights insists on an actively 'insane' status in order for involuntary treatment to be continued. To insist on continued treatment when an individual is well (the essence of continuing remission for patients with schizophrenia, for example) may be seen as contravening this approach. The rising use of tribunals or judges' decisions in difficult cases, and the increasing legislation surrounding the processes of community care, can be expected to continue. Nevertheless, a coherent community care policy must also embrace those (such as the severely ill) lacking insight, and the development of a humane community treatment order will be essential to this process.

Funding

The switch from short-term solutions, based on the random use of cheaper voluntary sector or 'skill mix reviews', will require more defined capitation formulae. The information technology required to run this will in itself be costly and will put patients at risk of breach of confidentiality given the availability of such data. Health priorities will have to be discussed both locally and nationally, since the impact of 'untoward incidents' (the main engine in the 1990s for increased provision) is bound to wane. The cost of new medication, which is likely to result in reduced demand for hospital beds, may give rise to complex economic arguments. Protecting mental health funds from the depredations of the acute sector, with its much 'sexier' image of high-tech medicine, without simultaneously divorcing mental health from the health care agenda in general, will require considerable political skills.

The social/health divide

The co-ordination of such services has long been a necessity, and is already accepted in certain localities. The main impediments relate to legislation and to professional factors, particularly at the senior managerial level. The size of any co-ordinated body may also be unwieldy, and its responsiveness (or robustness) to political intervention may impair its effectiveness. Nevertheless, if community care for the mentally ill has any one message to give, it is that the notions of 'health' and 'social' care are indivisible. As terms they are probably out of date but their full integration, at the individual, local and national levels, which will involve the sacrifice of cherished theories, must be a priority.

6. Getting Older: Epidemiology, Policy Dilemmas and Policy Trade-Offs

Siân Griffiths and
Jonathan McWilliam

For those working in the public sector, the demands for health and social care for older people are all too obvious. In this chapter we will sketch out some of the challenges – demographic, epidemiological, economic – and some of the dilemmas – funding, choice and rationing of care – which are involved. The problems of an ageing society are common to many cultures, and the solutions will need to address the same issues, making compromises and trade-offs in reaching decisions.

The challenge of demography and epidemiology

A number of demographic and epidemiological factors will combine over the next ten to twenty years to ensure that the issue of caring for older people remains at the forefront of the health policy agenda. First, the number of older people in Britain (defined arbitrarily as sixty-five years and over) is increasing, particularly the very elderly (those defined as over eighty-five).[64] Second, and perhaps more importantly from an economic point of view, the number of older people will increase as a proportion of the adult population. Those in the fifteen to sixty-four age group are estimated to increase in number by only 3 per cent between 1989 and 2026, compared with a projected 62 per cent rise in the eighty-five plus age group.[70] In other words, this less economically active group will grow rapidly, relative to the more economically active section of the population. A similar pattern will be seen in most western societies, and this will tend to increase per capita demand for expenditure on health services.

A number of social factors will also have a bearing on the type and style of services demanded. For example, at birth, females can expect to live between five and six years longer than males; hence women will continue to outnumber men as the population ages, the effect becoming more marked with increasing age. Another key trend is the increase in the proportion of elderly people living alone, which rose from 22 per cent in 1962 to 36 per cent in 1989.[71] The profile of carers of elderly people will also shift, so that carers themselves will be more likely to be elderly as the proportion of people aged eighty-five and over increases. The ethnic mix of elderly people will also change, with the proportion of the elderly from all ethnic minorities increasing. The impact of these demographic factors is difficult to determine, but one vital point for policy makers to grasp is that elderly people are a heterogeneous and constantly changing group, and that all policy directed towards them will therefore need to be flexible if it is to meet their evolving needs.

Turning from demography to epidemiology, although it is true that many elderly people live active, healthy lives, many others experience health problems which increase in frequency and severity as the patients grow older. Many of the health problems common in people aged over seventy-five result from chronic disabling conditions which – unlike, for example, provision of elective surgery in younger age groups – do not lend themselves to simple policy options. Common disabling conditions include neurological diseases such as strokes, dementia and Parkinson's disease; cardiovascular conditions such as angina and heart failure;

respiratory diseases such as bronchitis and emphysema; muscle and joint conditions such as arthritis; and other common problems such as incontinence. As the population ages, the prevalence of all these conditions is likely to increase. Since these common diseases are both chronic and incurable, the demand for services is likely to continue to spiral upwards.

Rates of acute illness, chronic illness and disability all tend to rise steeply with increasing age, and, coupled with the demographic factors outlined above, will continue to fuel demand. The impact of these trends will translate into increasing demand for institutional care before death. The proportion of the population aged sixty-five to seventy-four in institutional care is currently one per cent, rising sharply to 25 per cent for those aged over eighty-five.[72]

Not all sub-groups within the population have the same expectations for health and illness. There are marked inequalities between social class groups: those in manual social classes experience proportionally worse health, greater disability and earlier death than their contemporaries in professional classes. Thus those groups which are least able to pay for and direct their own care are the very ones who are likely to need it the most.

At the same time, there is little convincing evidence to suggest that the duration and severity of ill health before death are decreasing. The period preceding death is a time of intense resource utilisation. Debates about levels of clinical intervention continue to highlight the ongoing dilemma of quantity versus quality of life. We will develop this theme later in the chapter. So a gradual increase in demand for health care can be predicted on the basis of demographic and epidemiological evidence. Hence the key dilemma which society now faces is that of how to meet these growing needs with the limited resources available.

Economic challenges

It is difficult to generalise about older people; the category incorporates a diverse population across the 65 to 105 age group, and covers the full range of economic statuses. While many elderly people are financially independent and continue to generate wealth, in general old age tends to be a time of husbanding the resources accumulated in previous decades, and of living on a lower level of income. The census shows that older people in Britain are less economically active than their younger counterparts, and that the proportion of older people who are economically active is gradually decreasing.[73]

Reduced economic activity, particularly among men, seems to result from the interplay of several related factors. These include:

- structural factors – financial expectations based on the use of private pensions, state pensions and social security entitlements, rather than paid work
- demand for labour – the expectation of working into old age has gradually decreased; a depressed labour market and the timing of retirement to ensure eligibility for the state pension have contributed to this
- ill-health and disability – both increase gradually with age. Ill health is a key factor in the decision to retire.

Income in older age may come from a variety of sources, such as paid employment, pensions, or savings and investments. There is evidence to suggest that, overall, elderly people are gradually becoming better off. However, there are also indications that elderly people in Britain are potentially less well-off than their counterparts in Europe and North America. Moreover, some elderly people in Britain are still defined as living in poverty or on the margins of poverty. Victor has summarised the situation as follows:

Approximately 25 per cent of those aged sixty-five plus have an income at or below supplementary benefit rates and a further 44 per cent live on the margins of poverty (within 40 per cent of the poverty level). Within the elderly population it is the very old (people aged over eighty), women, those living alone, those from manual occupations and the disabled, who are most at risk of poverty in later life.[74]

Poverty lies at the root of many of the inequalities in health status. Hence the scale of poverty poses a major challenge to those concerned with redressing inequitable health status and service provision for the elderly.

Funding challenges – how should health care for the elderly be paid for?

Having recognised elderly people's greater need for health care, the question of funding – both current and future –

must be faced. There is a limited number of funding options available and these pose a variety of policy dilemmas. The main options for funding are:

1. Private care

Private health care can be purchased only by consumers with independent purchasing power. Although there are elderly people who have the resources to pay for their own care as needs arise, many elderly people have low levels of income. Thus, unless the state undertook to top-up income, a system funded solely from private sources would exacerbate existing inequalities in health and discriminate against the most vulnerable.

2. Insurance systems

Insurance schemes tend to work against the interests of elderly people, in that insurers classify old age as a period of high risk. Premiums are high and exclusions are many: home nursing, mental illness services and long-term care are frequently not covered. It would, however, be possible for the state to change the rules to extend coverage.

3. Direct taxation, including National Insurance contributions

In systems where income on earnings is taxed, elderly people, on the whole, will contribute less because their income is lower. On the other hand they will tend to utilise the most health care. This creates several difficulties. First, there may be a shortfall between income from taxation and expenditure, thus increasing the potential need for rationing (see below). Second, direct taxation tends to be divisive in that today's main funders are not today's main beneficiaries. This might lead to resentment among younger wage earners, who may perceive themselves as taxed excessively to meet others' needs. There may also be a reluctance among elderly people to use services which they see as based on handouts from other groups. Psychologically this conflict is dealt with via the popular myth that the National Insurance contributions which one makes during working life are somehow held by the government to pay for one's health needs in old age. This, of course, is not the case; in times of financial hardship it also leads to the problem of elderly people being denied the care for which they believe they have already paid. A recent example of this in Britain is the resentment caused by reduction of the state-funded long-term care to which many elderly people feel entitled.

4. Patient charges

Charging patients for specific services, such as eye tests or prescribed medication, involves striking a difficult balance between the increase in revenue expected, the administrative costs incurred and the effect of suppressed demand. Although elderly people are often exempt from such charges, the effect of levying them may well be to deter the elderly from seeking care, thereby exacerbating the existing unmet need within this group.

5. Lotteries/appeals/charitable donations

These methods of raising money have the disadvantage of being uncertain in yield, difficult and expensive to administer and unlikely to generate enough income to make an appreciable difference. The National Lottery has shown that it is often those with least resources who play on a regular basis, thus exacerbating the needs of the worse off.

Given the various models for funding health care, the dilemma of how best to finance the care of elderly people continues to be debated. This is not least because of the problematic interface between health and social care. The introduction of community care and care plans has highlighted the different funding structures for health and social care. It has also highlighted the arbitrary differences resulting from the need to make local decisions on such issues as eligibility criteria. With health and social care inexorably linked, decisions regarding appropriate forms of care often have more to do with the power of persuasion than with the needs of the individual. One solution would be to integrate health and social care, particularly the resources available for care of the elderly. However, while this might free up some resources, we must also make clear that the state is unlikely to be able to meet all the needs of the elderly, and make explicit the existing plurality of funding sources. The level of contribution from the state will be an issue for debate. In all western societies, state funding plays a key role in providing for health care, although Britain is unusual in not relying on a greater mix of public or private funding.

Grey politics:
the challenge from the consumers

While the number of elderly in the population grows and their relative poverty increases, they are becoming increasingly vocal in articulating their demands for rights through the 'grey movement'. Their central aim is to mobilise the sleeping giant of elderly people's political power so as to secure a better deal in society, if necessary via the ballot box. To date, success has been mixed, but it may well increase with the growing proportion of elderly people in the population.

Increasing use of the health service by elderly people is already visible, with consultation rates in general practice continuing to rise steadily, and with each individual calling on the service more often.[75] Some GPs say they are used more as an impersonal service, expected to be fully available around the clock, than as a personal service used sparingly. The reasons for this change are complex, but one clear trend is the increase in consumer demand. Consequences include the introduction of GP co-ops to deal with increased out-of-hours demands.

One could argue that the growth of the elderly population increases the demand for health care. Ageism is seen by many as unacceptable within health care, and refusal of treatment on the grounds of age alone is problematic. For example, decisions about who should receive coronary artery by-pass surgery need to be set against the patient's ability to benefit from the intervention, rather than simply on age criteria alone. An older patient may well be more likely to have co-morbidity, and thus age becomes an implicit rather than explicit criterion in decision making.

Another perspective on the relevance of care comes from patients themselves. The benefits of, say, surgical interventions, must be regarded not only from the perspective of the clinician, but also from that of patients. Work in American has shown that when men are given information about the consequences of prostate surgery they often choose to avoid the operation. Resistance to ageist policies is led by elderly people themselves and puts the issue of consumer choice once more at centre stage.

An increase in consumer choice can, however, work both ways. If all treatments, no matter how invasive, are offered to a sick person of any age (or, in the case of acute or serious illness, to their family as proxy decision-makers) life may be prolonged in the face of pain or discomfort. Fear of loss of dignity at the end of life has led to the increased use of the advanced directive or living wills, designed to exercise consumer choice when the consumer cannot be consulted. Similarly, the need for quality rather than quantity of life may lead older people to refuse interventions.

Other ethical dilemmas: the End of Life

Some countries have liberal policies regarding the provision of a range of choices to individuals and their families, including euthanasia. In Britain, where more and more invasive and expensive interventions are often carried out in the last weeks of an individual's life, this is a hotly contested issue. For similar reasons, life is also maintained by measures such as artificial feeding when the chances of improvement are minute. It is as if the concepts of valuing life, anti-ageism and defensive practice, combine to produce a result which is at best unbalanced, and at worst inhumane.

In the context of growing numbers of elderly and of growing numbers of available interventions, it may be appropriate to reappraise the role of the state in health care. The dilemma of providing for an ageing population with state resources which have diminished in real terms, raises the question of how much the state should be involved in health care provision.

State involvement in both the regulation and the provision of health care exists, in varying degrees, across the international arena. There are a number of arguments about the appropriate level of state involvement. These are summarised below.

The well-being of the many

Some things are considered to be so important to the well-being of society as a whole that they are provided for by the state as a priority and not left to the discretion of the individual. Typical examples include protection of society from communicable diseases (through immunisation and through public health laws to protect the environment and combat contagion); maintenance of a healthy work-force (via, for example, occupational health services) and, less prominent in the modern day, the need for a fit fighting force when required (the historical roots of the health visiting service). The majority of services provided under this heading tend to benefit children and adults. Elderly people are less likely to benefit.

Politico–philosophical factors

Our view of what constitutes a civilised society varies over time. First, there is the need to strike the right balance between the discretion of the individual and the discretion of the state (a pendulum which has swung towards the individual over the past two decades). The state acts as a utilitarian redistributor of resources so that those resources are shared as fairly as possible to achieve the greatest good for the greatest number. Second, there is the concept of human rights, which expects the provision of minimum standards for all members of a society. Those who are judged unable to provide for themselves are provided with a basic level of care.

Given the economic circumstances of many elderly people, and their consequent lack of discretion, the majority will benefit from input by the state, especially if utilitarian redistribution occurs. Conversely, the majority of older people would tend to fare worse where individuals are expected to buy their own health care within a market.

Economic and market factors

The state plays a number of roles, relating to economic and market factors, on behalf of elderly people. Each of these roles stems from a common source: namely, the inability of the free market to provide elderly people with the type of service deemed necessary in western societies. The various roles are as follows:

- Externalities
  The free market fails to take account of the cumulative benefit gained by society from procedures such as immunisation. Immunisation is generally provided free to the individual in order to encourage uptake. For example, older people are provided with flu vaccine free of charge to prevent them contracting the virus, and to preclude possible hospital admissions.

- Caring externality
  Western societies become concerned when an individual is ill but cannot afford treatment. In these circumstances, care tends to be financed or subsidised either by the state or by charities.

- Public goods
  While some forms of health care – such as elective surgery – could be subject to the traditional relationship of supply and demand, the relationship breaks down for other forms of care such as preventive interventions. With regard to elderly people, the question might arise as to who should pay for a programme of home safety improvements, given that the individuals who will benefit will never be detected.

- Monopolies
  Large hospitals can act as monopolies, either because they are the only geographical alternative, or because economies of scale allow them to undercut competitors. Once a monopoly is established, the price of the service

can be increased irrespective of the cost of providing it. Geographical monopolies are more easily established with regard to elderly people because of the difficulties they have with mobility. For example, monopolies can occur even in rural primary care where there is little choice, as well as in areas of the country served by single large hospitals.

- Empowerment

  A doctor generally knows more about diagnosis and treatment than the patient. This gives the doctor the opportunity to boost prices and denies the consumer choice. This effect can be offset in a number of ways: by paying GPs a capitation fee, rather than fees per service, as in Britain and the Health Maintenance Organisation systems; by paying consultants a salary rather than fees for service; by allowing easy access to second opinions; and by making objective information readily available to patients. It is not clear whether older people are particularly disadvantaged by lack of knowledge, but reduced mobility and lack of familiarity with modern information technology are unlikely to act in their favour. The tendency for older people to suffer from multiple conditions and to have simultaneous health and social care needs is a further disadvantage as it adds to the complexity of the issues which they would need to unravel as consumers.

- Merit wants

  Some things are valued so highly by society that they

should be provided for publicly rather than left to the vagaries of the market. Education is a good example, and it is often argued that a basic level of health care also falls into this category.

- Uncertainty of demand
  It is difficult to predict illness and to know as an individual whether you have provided adequately for the worst eventuality. The general solution is to pool the risk, and this is the basis both of state health care and private insurance companies. The difficulties with insurance systems have been discussed above.

The overall level of state involvement depends on a balance of these factors. There is a variety of roles for the state to play in regulating the market, in particular, as the honest broker and provider of objective information. This can help uninformed consumers to make sound choices. There is also an important role for the state in monitoring the quality, as well as in controlling prices, of the monopolies.

The state also becomes involved as supplier or agent for a basic range of services to meet the needs of the least well-off. This role may expand, as it does in Britain, to the state itself acting as a service which seeks to manage financial risk, control quality, seek economies of scale and provide the services which benefit the population as a whole, rather than only the individual.

New technologies

New treatments and new equipment are constantly being developed. A proportion of these will inevitably benefit elderly people. Although some new treatments offer greater efficiencies overall, many are either simply more expensive than the older treatments, or offer a new therapy for previously untreatable conditions. New technologies therefore present dilemmas to policy makers. Assuming that the new treatment is clinically effective, most of the dilemmas revolve around affordability, whether in the public or private sector. The prospect of new and expensive treatments for common conditions such as dementia pose particular challenges: who can best afford the new treatment – the individual, the insurer or the state?

New technologies can also stretch established policy in unexpected ways. The advent, for example, of telemedicine or of cheaper, smaller, more portable equipment, can open up the provision of services in peripheral sites, changing the whole character of a service. This may improve, for example, elderly people's access to treatments in health centres rather than treatment in distant specialist centres. The challenge for policy makers is, where possible, to keep abreast of new developments and to retain a flexible approach to designing services.

Rationing

In the face of limited resources rationing is inevitable. There is simply not enough money to pay for health needs, whether services are funded from the public or the private purse. The main issues for elderly people are the following:

Who should ration – the individual or the state?

In a perfect world the consumer would choose the goods and services he or she requires. In practice, rationing tends to occur at two levels, conducted by two distinct agents: first, by the state, with varying degrees of individual involvement, and second, by the individual for private care.

A major policy issue is how to involve elderly people in the state's decisions. This involvement can be divided into two types, based on the rights, versus the responsibilities, of the individual. Turning first to the rights-based rationale for involvement, the state acknowledges that it is acting as a proxy for consumers and that consumers therefore have a right to be involved in the decision-making process. Elderly people may be involved in this process in a number of ways, such as through established special interest organisations such as Age Concern; through statutory patient watchdog groups such as the Community Health Council; or through especially constituted panels comprising elderly people, their representatives and their carers. Some attempts to ration services involve canvassing the views of the whole population. Initiatives of this type, such as the work carried out in Oregon, have met with mixed success and tend to reflect the beliefs of the majority at the expense of minority groups. It may be that mass canvassing of public opinion would act against the interests of elderly people in this way.

The timing and depth of consumer involvement also varies widely, ranging from detailed involvement right through the policy making process, to brief consultation on a fixed number of options. Consumer groups favour more involvement rather than less, and this presents state providers with a number of challenges, including their willingness and ability to make the process more open. Further challenges include the increased workload owing to the involvement of people in the process and, perhaps most of all, that of balancing the needs of one care group against the needs of others. In a climate of pressure on public spending, how can the merits of treatments for older people be compared with treatments for children if only one can be afforded?

Consumers are involved in the rationing debate at the ballot box. The public votes indirectly for the resource-base of state health services. There are major policy dilemmas for political parties, which have to weigh their desire to develop public services with the current unpopularity of direct funding from the taxpayer.

Public involvement may also be based on the notion of the public as a responsible consumer of resources. Responsibility may be articulated in two main ways: incentivising responsible consumption and responsible lifestyle. Policies aimed at increasing consumption include schemes to issue each person at birth with some form of health care token or voucher which can be redeemed against services throughout life, as and when required. This method has the theoretical advantage of allowing consumers to choose the care they need. Policies to incentivise lifestyle include penalising, or denying an individual access to care if he or she exhibits behaviour damaging to health, such as smoking and drinking to excess.

More sophisticated methods combine incentivised

consumption and incentivised lifestyle. In managed care, for example, the individual pays for a package of care programmes which range from health promotion through to treatment and care for a given range of conditions. This method therefore attempts to involve the consumer in constraining both demand for the service (via a healthy lifestyle) and supply of the services (via treatment protocols). Each of these ideas runs into a number of problems:

- Who determines what constitutes a good or bad lifestyle when evidence is inconclusive?
- Is access to health care a moral issue?
- How do consumers weigh up how to provide in the present for intangible questions such as how long they will live, how sick they might become and how much treatment they might need in the future?
- Lack of consumer knowledge.
- The costs of administration.
- How to deal with the under-insured.
- The distaste society would have for leaving those who had either spent all their tokens or those who had smoked too much with no service at all.

From the specific perspective of elderly people, we could also add the fear of running out of credit in later years, and the difficulty of knowing what resources to husband for a possible long and expensive final illness. Various amendments can be made to soften incentivised systems to meet some of these objections, but these inevitably bring us back towards more straightforward state care.

Rationing the supply side

Issuing tokens is a means of controlling the demand side of the health care equation. Other attempts to control demand include cash-limited public expenditure, introducing charges for certain services and allowing only specific groups such as poorer people access to the service. Policies may also be directed at controlling the supply side of the equation. Some of the current means of doing this are:

Clinical rationing

Clinical criteria can be used to judge which services will be available in state-run care and which services will not. In Britain in recent years the state has devolved this decision to health authorities, each of which covers between 500,000 and 1,000,000 people. Methods used may include: purchasing only treatments of known clinical effectiveness; comparing the cost and quality of similar treatments and supplying the cheaper; and obliging clinicians to work to, but not beyond, agreed treatment protocols.

Reducing the size of the state's stake

This form of rationing chips away at the block of state provision and moves whole areas of care into the private/charging sector. Examples of this kind of proposal include: limiting the breadth of services covered by the state by not providing services such as cosmetic surgery or IVF; decreasing the state's spend on social care while transferring the costs to user and carer; charging for the non-acute aspects of care, via, for example, hotel costs during recuperation following surgery; shortening the duration of care in the state's facilities, for example, by introducing more ambulatory care and reduced hospital stays; and increasing charges for prescriptions and for services such as dental care. Once again, these changes will tend to affect the less well-off elderly consumer disproportionately, especially as elderly people are the slowest to recover and the group who benefit most from longer state care.

The dilemma of social care

Some would argue that the existence of the welfare state (aided and abetted by the medical profession) has 'medicalised' growing old to the extent that old age itself is now seen as a disease. Placing the responsibility for decision-making and funding back with the consumer can be seen as an attempt to 'demedicalise' the care of older people. This has happened recently in British social care. Although this can also be seen as a pure cost-cutting exercise, it is worth reflecting on the particular dilemmas thrown up by social care.

Social care presents particular dilemmas to policy makers. These dilemmas concern principally older people who are most in need of social care. The main issues are as follows:

- At what point do individual responsibilities end and those of the state begin?
  Social care is harder to define than health care. It differs from health care in that it merges into, or is similar to, the care provided within many families. It does not necessarily involve trained professionals and it does not call for the same degree of specialisation or technological

support as health care. Delineating a clear cut-off point between self-provision and care by the state or charities is more difficult than in health care. Nonetheless, elderly people do have key social needs – such as shelter, food, and, in many cases, increasing assistance with walking and washing – which need to be met.

- If it is difficult to fund health care, how can society ever hope to fund social care?
  Although western societies are unwilling to leave individuals with insufficient social care, a tougher line is taken regarding state provision than in health care. As public spending controls become more stringent, the threshold at which the state will intervene becomes even more 'high and tight'. A whole series of measures is introduced to ration state support, including a detailed assessment of needs, means-testing, charging and capping the total state spend, while simultaneously stimulating the private sector to provide alternatives.

The conservation of capital within families has become a controversial issue in the social care debate in recent years. A pattern has emerged in which elderly people often sell their homes to pay for residential care in their last year of life. Older people, many of whom believe that the state should provide this care in total, feel they are forced to cash in the inheritance they had hoped to pass on. Families also feel cheated and are reluctant to acknowledge that the road to inheritance lies in providing care within the family. This is a clear example of policy incentivising particular forms of social change. Should the policy continue, it will be interesting to see where the balance between private residential care and care within the family is set.

The tactics of rationing health care

Rationing decisions can be made more or less openly. Recent years have witnessed what could be seen as a process of rationing by stealth, in which an open debate on the need to ration health care is avoided, and the service offered by the state is gradually reduced. A more cynical view is that the provision of low quality state care provides a hidden incentive to the consumer to seek alternatives outside the state-run sector. A policy of openness is greatly to be preferred, as it treats the electorate as adults, and helps society as a whole to decide on difficult issues. It would be in the interests of elderly people to open up the debate, as their need for support from the more economically active section of the population is crucial. The growing extent of the problem owing to demographic factors alone needs to be understood by everyone. Only then can the electorate balance the costs and benefits of policies such as reducing public spending on health care.

Broader health issues and the broader political agenda

So far we have discussed future provision of health services. In reality, the health of elderly people depends on much more than health services alone. Some of the main additional factors are as follows:

- Environmental factors
  Many agencies play a part in providing a safe and secure
  environment, from the Environmental Health
  Departments of local authorities, to the local police force.
  Co-ordination is vital, and the recent initiatives in Britain
  to strengthen partnerships between government
  departments are welcome.

- Lifestyle factors and health promotion
  It is better to promote health than to treat disease. For
  many years within the NHS, efforts to help people make
  healthy choices have taken a back seat compared with the
  necessity of providing treatment today. For young people,
  the choices of today can cast long shadows forward to
  result in disease in old age. It is becoming clearer that
  changes in exercise and diet can decrease the incidence of
  common conditions such as heart disease, strokes and
  cancers of the digestive tract, as well as staving off many
  chronic conditions which are exacerbated by excess
  weight and poor mobility.

These factors would also make a real impact on the
problems of financing health care. The issue for policy
makers and politicians is to look beyond today's crises and to
find ways of investing in, for example, health-promoting
food policies, or in combating anti-health lobby groups such
as the tobacco industry. Both America and Britain have
begun to shift their approaches, and the launch of Our
Healthier Nation, in particular, emphasises the cross-
government departmental flavour of the task. Yet there is a

long way to go before broader health issues and a preventive approach can take the key place in policy that logic demands.

Summary

The main trends which will influence policy in the next millenium are listed below. Where appropriate, conclusions have been drawn and recommendations made for action.

- Although demand will continue to rise and treatment possibilities will broaden, the ability of society to pay for services could well diminish in proportion.
- Increasing demand is fuelled by a mixture of demographic, epidemiological and social factors, including increased consumer activity.
- The advantages of retaining a large state sector input in the care of elderly people are overwhelming. Yet, where societies are unwillling to deprive elderly people of a basic service, rationing in this sector is inevitable.
- It is likely that the core of state provision will operate on utilitarian lines.
- An open public debate is required on three main topics:
  i) The mechanism for rationing.
  ii) How to ensure a humane and dignified end to life.
  iii) How to set a balanced level of public spending.
- Controls on the supply-side of the equation will increase, governed by clinical effectiveness and treatment protocols.
- A lively private sector will continue to flourish, and its input in health care is likely to grow. There will be a

gradual increase in the proportion of elderly people who are willing and able to select private services.

- The trend towards self-sufficiency in social care is likely to continue.
- An 'honest broker' function is required by the public, by government and by the private sector, to provide unbiased information to assist these debates.
- Concentration on health promotion, disease prevention and a multi-agency approach to health care could play an important part in controlling demand.

Notes

Introduction

1   Duff Cooper, *Talleyrand*, Phoenix Giant edition, London, 1997, p.228.

2   Ferdinand Mount offers the idea of a 'market-plus' approach to these questions. See his article 'A niche market for the Tories', *Sunday Times*, News Review section, 21 September 1997, p.4.

3   Sir Douglas Black, *Inequalities of Health*, Department of Health and Social Security, London, 1980; For a view from the Child Poverty Action Group see Carey Oppenheim and Lisa Harker, *Poverty the Facts*, revised third edition, London, 1996. A corrective is Norman Dennis, *The Invention of Permanent Poverty*, The Child Poverty Action Group Institute of Economic Affairs Health and Welfare Unit, London, 1997 and Richard Pryke, *Taking the Measure of Poverty, A Critique of Low-Income Statistics: Alternative Estimates and Policy Implications*, IEA Health and Welfare Unit, London, 1995; also, Charles Murray et al., *Charles Murray and the Underclass: The Developing Debate*, Institute of Economic Affairs Health & Welfare Unit, London, 1996, in which Alan Buckingham offers 'A Statistical Update'. See also David J. Smith (ed.), *Understanding the Underclass*, Policy Studies Institute, London, 1992, which includes David Green's 'Liberty, Poverty and the Underclass. A classical-liberal approach to public policy', pp.68–87.

4   See British Medical Association Health Policy and Economic Research Unit report, *Options for Funding Health Care*, London, BMA, October 1997. For the alternative, see David G. Green, 'From National Health Monopoly to National Health Guarantee', in David Gladstone (ed.) *How to Pay for Health Care: Public and Private Alternatives*, Institute of Economic Affairs Health and Welfare Unit, London, 1997. Also, David G. Green, 'Future funding of NHS "monopoly"', Letter to *The Times*, 9 October 1997, p.21

5   *Independent Perspectives on Health and Social Care*, Independent Health care Association, London, 1996; William Rees-Mogg, 'Beds, not trolleys. Britain is underfunding health care especially in the private sector,' *The Times*, 27 February 1997, p.18, and 'Why the NHS is the sick man of Europe', *The Times*, 6 October 1997, p.20.

6   Duff Cooper, op. cit., pp. 303–5.

The Cost of Caring: A Tale of Innocence and Experience

7   *Health News*, King's Fund, London, 1997.

8   A. Williams, 'Rationing health care by age', *British Medical Journal*, 314, 1997, pp.820–22.

9   G. Rivett, *From Cradle to Grave: Health care and the health service*, King's Fund, London, forthcoming January 1998; p.110.

10   D. W. Light, 'The real ethics of rationing', *British Medical Journal*, 315,1997, pp.112-15.

11   See B. New and J. Le Grand, *Rationing in the NHS: Principles & pragmatism*, King's Fund, London, 1996.

12   N. Timmins, *The Five Giants: A biography of the welfare state*, HarperCollins, London, 1995, p.101.

13   A. Coote, 'The views of the public should be directly taken into account in making rationing decisions', in B. New, (ed.), *Rationing: Talk and action in health care*, British Medical Journal/King's Fund, London, 1997.

14   See the series 'Promoting Patient Choice', King's Fund, 1996–97.

15   J. Spiers, '"Only a Novel!"': Jane Austen, hypertext, and the story of patient power', in M. Marinker (ed.), *Sense and Sensibility in Health Care*, British Medical Journal, London, 1996.

16   V. Entwistle, I. Watt *et al*. 'The media and the message', in M. Marinker (ed.), *Sense and Sensibility in Health Care*, British Medical Journal, London, 1996.

17   Michael Young suggested a voucher system for GPs as long ago as 1989. Vouchers are discussed in J. Le Grand and W. Bertlett (eds.) *Quasi-Markets and Social Policy*, Macmillan, Basingstoke, 1994, pp. 7–10.

18   H. Goodare, 'The possibilities for direct patient involvement in rationing decisions', in B. New (ed.), *Rationing: Talk and action in health care*, British Medical Journal/King's Fund, 1997.

Evidence-based Medicine: A Consensus Dream or a Practical Reality?

19   *Tidal Wave, New Technology and the NHS*, King's Fund, London, 1992.

20   T. A. Brennan *et al*, 'Incidence of Adverse Events and Negligence in Hospitalised Patients: Results of the Harvard Medical Practice Study 1', *New England Journal of Medicine*, Vol.324, 1991, pp.370–76.

21   M. Baum, Letter in the *British Medical Journal*, Vol. 282, 1981, pp.68–69.

22   *Tidal Wave, New Technology and the NHS*, op. cit.

23   D. Saunders, A. Coulter and K. McPherson, *Variations in Hospital Admission Rates: A Review of the Literature*, Kings Fund, London, 1989.

24   See M. M. Rosenthal, *The Incompetent Doctor: Behind Closed Doors*, Open University Press, Buckingham, 1995.

Healthcare Funding and Outcomes: Will Your NHS Insurance Cover Meet Your Needs?

25   NHS Executive, *Changing the Internal Market*, EL97, 33, Department of Health, Leeds, 1997.

26   *Department of Health Central Health Outcomes Unit*, London,
      Department of Health, 1994.

27   *The National Health Service: A service with ambitions*, HMSO, London, 1996.

28   NHS Executive, *Changing the Internal Market*, op.cit.

29   National Confidential Enquiry into Perioperative Deaths, *Report of the National
      Confidential Enquiry into Perioperative Deaths 1993/94*, NCEPOD, London, 1996.

Shifting the Boundaries: Partnerships in Total Health Care

30   Thanks are due to colleagues who commented on earlier drafts of this chapter,
      including Nick Allen, Andrew Mortimore, Simon Tanner and Ian Marriott at the
      Health Authority, Chris Ham at HSMC Birmingham and members of the SMF health
      study group, chaired by Rick Nye.

31   Locality commissioning is used here to refer to the devolution of a wide range of
      responsibilities of the Health Authority, including the delegation of funds for purchasing
      hospital and community health services, to groups of GP practices organised on a
      geographical basis. There is a wide variety of differing models which exist within this
      broad concept.

32   Total purchasing refers to an extended version of fundholding introduced on a limited
      basis by the NHS Executive from 1995 onwards, starting in Bromsgrove, Worth Valley,
      Runcorn and Berkshire. Again, a variety of forms have been adopted but generally they
      involve the devolution of a budget which covers emergency care and other services
      beyond the scope of standard fundholding, thus placing fundholders more firmly into
      the arena of 'strategic' commissioning and the overall balance of priorities and resources.

33.   Managed care can be better described than defined. In this context we mean systems of
      health care funding, typically in America, which attempt to control expenditure through
      creating financial incentives for cost-effective resource use by clinicians. This involves
      management protocols usually based on care pathways, disease management 'packages',
      utilisation review and a variety of other techniques. It is the opposite of 'fee for service'
      remuneration as it usually relies on a fixed 'capitation' fee for managing the health care
      of a defined population.

34   R. Robinson and J. Le Grand (eds.), *Evaluating the NHS Reforms*, Kings Fund, London,
      1994.

35   J. Dixon and H. Glennerster, 'What do we know about fundholding in General
      Practice?', *British Medical Journal*, 311, 1995, pp.727-730.

36   The evidence which suggests this is largely anecdotal and because of the difficulties of
      using historic activity data and the problems of taking into account trends in casemix, is
      often incomplete. A study in Southampton undertaken in 1996 compared the relative
      'purchasing power' for chargeable procedures of GP fundholders and non-fundholders.
      It concluded that changes in the balance of emergency (non-chargeable) and elective
      (chargeable) work had not been fully taken into account in setting fundholder budgets
      in previous years. For an explanation of the methodology used, see the paper 'GPFH

Resource Allocation', 7 January 1997, available from the Health Authority.

37　Adjustments to fundholder budgets were made by several health authorities, including Wiltshire and Cornwall, for similar reasons.

38　R. Robinson and J. Le Grand, 'Markets and Contracting in Health Care', IHPS Occasional Paper, Institute for Health Policy Studies, Southampton, 1994.

39　F. Honigsbaum, J. I. Richards and A. L. Lockett, *Priority Setting in Action*, Radcliffe Medical Press, Oxford, 1995.

40　BMJ (eds.), *Rationing in Action*, BMJ Publishing, London, 1993.

41　'Crash Test Dummies: Report on a locality commissioning simulation held in Wakefield', *Health Service Journal*, August 1997

42　Since the mid-1970s, 'growth' money allocated to the NHS has been differentially applied to health authorities around the country using various forms of weighted capitation formulae in order gradually to redress the regional inequities in funding which had arisen through supply-side factors, notably the concentration of teaching hospitals in London.

43　L. Mountford, address to a meeting at Richmond House of health economists working in the NHS, 19 March 1996.

44　The efficiency index is a figure used to indicate the overall performance of the NHS year on year in securing better value for money. It is the ratio of work done (activity) to resources used (expenditure). This is problematical because it focuses solely on outputs rather than outcomes, creating the mistaken impression that more is better. The index has also been skewed towards acute activity, which is easier to measure.

45　J. Appleby, *A measure of effectiveness?: A critical review of the NHS Efficiency Index*, National Association of Health Authorities and Trusts, Birmingham, 1996.

46　A. Harrison, 'Tomorrow's Hospital: The Future of the Acute Hospital in a Primary Care Led NHS', *Opinion*, 1, Bristol-Myers Squibb Pharmaceuticals, London, 1996.

47　C. Ham and J. Shapiro, 'Learning Curve', *Health Service Journal*, 18 January 1996, pp.24-25.

48　R. Robinson and A. Steiner, *The Performance of Managed Care: A Review of Evidence*, IHPS Research Paper, Southampton, 1996; J. Smith, M. Bamford, C. Ham, E. Scrivens and J. Shapiro, *Beyond fundholding: A mosaic of primary care led commissioning and provision in the West Midlands*, HSMC, Birmingham, 1997; C. Ham. 'Primary Managed Care in Europe', *British Medical Journal*, 314, 1997, p.457.

49　*Kaiser Permanente Healthwise Handbook*, Healthwise Incorporated, Idaho, 1996.

50　B. Kirkman-Liff, lecture on 'Commissioning Care: An American Perspective on the UK reforms', given at Manchester University, 1996.

The Future of Mental Health in a Community Setting

51　T. Groves, 'After the asylums', *British Medical Journal*, 300, 1990, pp.923-24.

52 K. Jones, *Asylums and After: A revised history of the mental health services from the early 18th century to the 1990s*, The Athlone Press, London, 1993.

53 Ibid.

54 See L. I. Stein and M. A. Test, 'Alternatives to mental hospital', *Archives of General Psychiatry*, 37, 1980, pp. 392–97; and T. Burns *et al*. 'A controlled trial of acute home-based psychiatric services', 1. Clinical and social outcome, *British Journal of Psychiatry* 163, 1993, pp.49–54.

55 J. Leff (ed.), *Care in the Community: Illusion or Reality?*, J. Wiley & Sons, London, 1997.

56 M. Wallace, 'The Forgotten Illness', articles reprinted from *The Times*, 1985/86.

57 See G. E. Berrios and H. Freeman (eds.), *150 Years of British Psychiatry 1841-1991*, Gaskell, London, 1991, especially D. Bennett 'The drive towards the community', Ch.21 pp. 321–32 and D. Tantam 'The anti-psychiatry movement', Ch.22, pp.333–47.

58 *The Report of the Inquiry into the Care and Treatment of Christopher Clunis*, HMSO, London, 1994.

59 M. Scazufca and E. Kuipers, 'Impact on women who care for those with schizophrenia', *Psychiatric Bulletin*, 21, 1997, pp.:469–71.

60 See J. Leff, *Care in the Community*, op. cit.

61 Ibid.

62 J. Repper, L. Sayce, S. Strong, J. Willmot and M. Haines, *Tall Stories from the Back Yard: A Survey of 'Nimby' Opposition to Community Mental Health Facilities, Experienced by Key Service Providers in England and Wales*, MIND, 1997.

63 *London's Mental Health: The Report to the King's Fund London Commission*, King's Fund, London, 1997. See especially 'Mental Health Services in London: Costs', pp.305-30.

64 See M. Deahl and T. Turner. 'General psychiatry in no-man's land', *British Journal of Psychiatry*, 171, 1997, pp.6-8, and P. Prosser *et al*, 'Mental Health, 'Burnout' and Job Satisfaction among Hospital and Community-Based Mental Health Staff', *British Journal of Psychiatry*, 169, 1996, pp.334-37

65 See *London's Mental Health*, op. cit.

66 'Introduction of Supervision Registers for Mentally Ill People from 1 April, 1994', *HSG*, 5, Department of Health, London, 1994.

67 For a review, see A. Maden. 'Correctional psychiatry', *Current Opinion in Psychiatry*, 9.6, 1996, pp.398-400.

68 *Making London Better*, Department of Health, DOH Publications Unit, Lancashire, 1993.

69 'Better off in the community?: The care of people who are seriously mentally ill', *House of Commons Health Committee, first report*, Vol. I, HMSO, London, 1994.

Getting Older: Epidemiology, Policy Dilemmas and Policy Trade-Offs

70   Health Advisory Service, *Services for people who are elderly: Addressing the balance*, HMSO, 1997.

71   Ibid.

72   Ibid.

73   C. R. Victor, *Health and Health Care in Later Life*, Open University Press, 1991.

74   Ibid.

75   OPCS, *Morbidity Statistics from General Practice 1991-92*, HMSO, 1995; *Morbidity Statistics from General Practice 1981-82*, HMSO, 1986 and *Morbidity Statistics from General Practice 1971-72*, HMSO, 1979.

Study Group Contributors

Ian Ayres, South West London Total Fundholding Project

Jessica Barrington, Social Market Foundation (Secretary)

Mark Bassett, NHS Executive Headquarters

Sue Botes, Health Visitors Association

Michael Dunning, The King's Fund

David Green, Institute of Economic Affairs, Health and Welfare Unit

Tony Hockley, Policy Analysis Centre

Tom Ling, Anglia University

Richard Marsh, Market Access

Matt Muijen, Sainsbury Centre for Mental Health

Roderick Nye, Social Market Foundation

Stephen Pollard, Social Market Foundation

Anne Richardson, Department of Health, Health Services Directorate

Leigh Richardson, Portsmouth Hospitals NHS Trust

Janice Robinson, The King's Fund

Claire Sweetman, Pfizer Ltd

Philip Watt, Pfizer Ltd

John Willman, Financial Times

John Young, Pfizer Ltd

Papers in Print

SMF Papers

Reports

Occasional Papers

7. Understanding 'Shock Therapy'
   Jeffrey Sachs
   £8.00

8. Recruiting to the Little Platoons
   William Waldegrave
   £6.00

9. The Culture of Anxiety: The Middle Class in Crisis
   Matthew Symonds
   £8.00

10. What is left of Keynes?
    Samuel Brittan, Meghnad Desai, Deepak Lal, Robert Skidelsky, Tom Wilson
    £8.00

11. Winning the Welfare Debate
    Peter Lilley (Introduction by Frank Field)
    £10.00

12. Financing the Future of the Welfare State
    Robert Skidelsky, Will Hutton
    £8.00

13. Picking Winners: The East Asian Experience
    Ian Little
    £8.00

14. Over-the-Counter Medicines
    Alan Maynard, Gerald Richardson
    £10.00

15. Pressure Group Politics in Modern Britain
    Riddell, Waldegrave, Secrett, Bazalgette, Gaines, Parminter
    £10.00

16. Design Decisions: Improving the Public Effectiveness of Public Purchasing
    Taylor, Fisher, Sorrell, Stephenson, Rawsthorn, Davis, Jenkins, Turner, Taylor
    £10.00

17. Stakeholder Society vs Enterprise Centre of Europe
    Robert Skidelsky, Will Hutton
    £10.00

18. Setting Enterprise Free
    Ian Lang
    £10.00

19. Community Values and the Market Economy
    John Kay
    £10.00

Other Papers

Local Government and the Social Market
George Jones
£3.00

Full Employment without Inflation
James Meade
£6.00

Memoranda

1. Provider Choice: 'Opting In' through the Private Finance Initiative
   Michael Fallon
   £5.00

2. The Importance of Resource Accounting
   Evan Davis
   £3.50

3. Why There is No Time to Teach:
   What is wrong with the National Curriculum 10 Level Scale
   John Marks
   £5.00

4. All Free Health Care Must be Effective
   Brendan Devlin, Gwyn Bevan
   £5.00

5. Recruiting to the Little Platoons
   William Waldegrave
   £5.00

6. Labour and the Public Services
   John Willman
   £8.00

7. Organising Cost Effective Access to Justice
   Gwyn Bevan, Tony Holland and Michael Partington
   £5.00

8. A Memo to Modernisers
    Ron Beadle, Andrew Cooper, Evan Davis, Alex de Mont,
    Stephen Pollard, David Sainsbury, John Willman
    £8.00

9. Conservatives in Opposition: Republicans in the US
    Daniel Finkelstein
    £5.00

10. Housing Benefit: Incentives for Reform
    Greg Clark
    £8.00

11. The Market and Clause IV
    Stephen Pollard
    £5.00

12. Yeltsin's Choice: Background to the Chechnya Crisis
    Vladimir Mau
    £8.00

13. Teachers' Practices: A New Model for State Schools
    Tony Meredith
    £8.00

14. The Right to Earn: Learning to Live with Top People's Pay
    Ron Beadle
    £8.00

15. A Memo to Modernisers II
    John Abbott, Peter Boone, Tom Chandos, Evan Davis, Alex de Mont, Ian Pearson MP,
    Stephen Pollard, Katharine Raymond, John Spiers
    £8.00

16. Schools, Selection and the Left
    Stephen Pollard
    £8.00

17. The Future of Long-Term Care
    Andrew Cooper, Roderick Nye
    £8.00

18. Better Job Options for Disabled People: Re-employ and Beyond
    Peter Thurnham
    £8.00

30. The Sex Change State
    Melanie Phillips
    £8.00

Trident Trust/
SMF Contributions to Policy

1. Welfare to Work: The *America Works* Experience
   Roderick Nye (Introduction by John Spiers)
   £10.00

2. Job Insecurity vs Labour Market Flexibility
   David Smith (Introduction by John Spiers)
   £10.00

3. How Effective is Work Experience?
   Greg Clark and Katharine Raymond (Foreword by Colin Cooke-Priest)
   £8.00

Hard Data

1. The Rowntree Inquiry and 'Trickle Down'
   Andrew Cooper, Roderick Nye
   £5.00

2. Costing the Public Policy Agenda: A week of the *Today* Programme
   Andrew Cooper
   £5.00

3. Universal Nursery Education and Playgroups
   Andrew Cooper, Roderick Nye
   £5.00

4. Social Security Costs of the Social Chapter
   Andrew Cooper, Marc Shaw
   £5.00

5. What Price a Life?
   Andrew Cooper, Roderick Nye
   £5.00

Centre for
Post-Collectivist Studies

1. Russia's Stormy Path to Reform
   Robert Skidelsky (ed.)
   £20.00

2. Macroeconomic Stabilisation in Russia: Lessons of Reforms, 1992–1995
   Robert Skidelsky, Liam Halligan
   £10.00

3. The End of Order
   Francis Fukuyama
   £9.50

Briefings

1. A Guide to Russia's Parliamentary Elections
   Liam Halligan, Boris Mozdoukhov
   £10.00